KETO BASICS

INCLUDES 50+ RECIPES

Your Guide to the Essentials of the Keto Diet—and How It Can Work for You!

KETO GUIDELINES

STARTER RECIPES

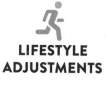

LIFESTYLE ADJUSTMENTS

Adams Media

New York London Toronto Sydney New Delhi

A adams media

Adams Media
An Imprint of Simon & Schuster, Inc.
57 Littlefield Street
Avon, Massachusetts 02322

First Adams Media trade paperback edition January 2019

ADAMS MEDIA and colophon are trademarks of Simon & Schuster.

For information about special discounts for bulk purchases, please contact Simon & Schuster Special Sales at 1-866-506-1949 or business@simonandschuster.com.

The Simon & Schuster Speakers Bureau can bring authors to your live event. For more information or to book an event contact the Simon & Schuster Speakers Bureau at 1-866-248-3049 or visit our website at www.simonspeakers.com.

Interior design by Stephanie Hannus
Interior images © 123RF; Getty Images

Manufactured in the United States of America

10 9 8 7 6 5 4 3

Library of Congress Cataloging-in-Publication Data has been applied for.

ISBN 978-1-5072-1009-3
ISBN 978-1-5072-1010-9 (ebook)

Contains material adapted from the following titles published by Adams Media, an Imprint of Simon & Schuster, Inc.: *The Everything® Guide to the Ketogenic Diet* by Lindsay Boyers, CHNC, copyright © 2015, ISBN 978-1-4405-8691-0; *The Everything® Ketogenic Diet Cookbook* by Lindsay Boyers, CHNC, copyright © 2017, ISBN 978-1-5072-0626-3; *The Everything® Big Book of Fat Bombs* by Vivica Menegaz, CTWFN, copyright © 2016, ISBN 978-1-4405-9675-9.

Contents

6: 50+ Ketogenic Recipes 151

Introduction

You've heard a lot about the benefits of the ketogenic diet. It can help you lose weight, reduce your risk of heart disease, lower your cholesterol, and so much more. But with *so* many rules and restrictions, where do you begin?

With the basics.

Keto Basics teaches you everything you need to know about the keto diet in a quick, easy-to-understand way. Wondering what you can eat? You'll discover the wide variety of delicious foods included in the keto diet. Confused about what ketosis is and what effect it has on your body? You'll find a clear explanation along with easy-to-follow guidelines. Are you concerned a low-carb, high-fat diet will just lead to weight gain? Not to worry! You'll learn why fat is your friend and how it can actually help you slim down. Plus, there are more than fifty delicious recipes that make it easy to stick to your keto guidelines!

You'll learn the ins and outs of keto-based eating. Once you have the information, you can tailor it specifically to your life. Maybe you want to calm chronic inflammation in your body or maybe you want to improve mental focus and boost your energy levels or maybe you're looking to shed those stubborn pounds you've been struggling with for years. Whatever your motives, with the *Keto Basics* covered you can be confident and successful in your diet decisions.

No matter what your reasons are for the ketogenic diet, this book is here to help you understand the keto diet and apply it to your life—easily and effectively.

1

Getting Started on the Keto Diet

As the name implies, the ketogenic diet is a diet plan that puts your body's innate intelligence to work by forcing your body to enter into a state of ketosis. You'll learn in the next chapter all about ketosis and how your body reacts to it, but for now know that ketosis is a metabolic state that can lead to significant weight loss when done properly. Your body already instinctively knows how to get into ketosis when you don't eat carbohydrates, but the point of the ketogenic diet is to force it to happen and keep it going for as long as you want. If you're interested in starting a ketogenic diet, the following information can help you get started.

What Is the Ketogenic Diet?

The ketogenic diet encourages you to get most of your calories from fat and to severely restrict carbohydrates. Unlike a typical low-carbohydrate diet the ketogenic diet is not a high-protein diet. Instead, it's a high-fat, moderate-protein, and low-carbohydrate diet. Although your exact macronutrient ratio will differ based on your individual needs, a typical nutritional ketogenic diet looks something like this:

Fat: 60 to 75 percent of calories

Protein: 15 to 30 percent of calories

Carbohydrates: 5 to 10 percent of calories

These are just general guidelines, but most people on a successful ketogenic diet fall somewhere in this range. In order to figure what you should be eating, you'll have to calculate your individual macronutrient ratios. As your diet progresses and your body begins to change, you may have to recalculate these numbers and make the proper adjustments to your diet plan.

Starting a Ketogenic Diet

If you're used to following a standard American diet—one in which most of your calories come from carbohydrates—a ketogenic diet is a major change, but it isn't so difficult that you won't be able to do it. All it takes is some commitment and preparation.

You have two choices when it comes to starting the keto diet: jump into it cold turkey or slowly wean yourself off carbohydrates, increasing your fat intake until your macronutrient ratios fall within your goal. When you go into it cold turkey, you're more likely to experience unpleasant carbohydrate withdrawal symptoms, so easing into it slowly is often the best bet for success.

Prepare Your Kitchen

Congratulations! You've decided to start the keto diet. That's the first step toward a healthy lifestyle change. Now that you've made the decision, you'll need to prepare your kitchen to set yourself up for success. This is a two-part process. First, you'll need to remove off-plan foods. Next, it's time to stock your refrigerator and pantry with the essentials. Sounds pretty easy, right?

If you live alone or with others who are also following a ketogenic diet, removing off-plan foods is simple. Go through your pantry and refrigerator and take out all the foods that don't fit into your diet plan. Don't forget to check the labels on your spices and dried herbs. Sometimes these contain sugar or other artificial ingredients that don't belong on a ketogenic diet. Donate unopened items to your local food pantry and toss the open ones in the trash.

If you're the only one in your household starting a ketogenic diet, this removal process is a little more complicated. Instead of donating or throwing out foods that are off-plan divide the pantry up. If possible put all ketogenic-approved foods in a separate cabinet and make it a point to go only in there and not even look in the off-plan cabinet. Dividing up the fridge might be even more difficult than dividing the pantry, but do the best you can to separate what you can eat from what you can't.

That's step one. The second part of preparing your kitchen is to stock up on all the essentials. It's imperative that you always have foods on hand that you can eat. If you don't, you're more likely to get to the point of being so hungry that you'll eat anything. Familiarize yourself with the essentials listed in the Appendix and keep your kitchen stocked with them at all times.

Carbohydrate Guides

Carbohydrate guides are a helpful tool to use with the ketogenic diet, especially when you're just starting out. Eating a low number of carbohydrates is essential when on the ketogenic diet. Many books are available that provide a list of foods and their carbohydrate count (as well as their calorie, protein, and fat content).

Some of these books categorize foods into high-carbohydrate, medium-carbohydrate, and low-carbohydrate lists. There are also several mobile apps that do the same thing.

Whatever method you choose, make sure you have your carbohydrate guide handy when you are food shopping so you can double-check what foods are allowed on the diet and which foods aren't. In a few pages you'll find a list of foods you should buy and foods you should avoid on the keto diet. As you get the hang of the diet, you won't need to check every single food before you purchase it, but it's still handy to have the guides easily accessible for those once-in-a-while foods that you're unsure about.

Ease Into It

When you're excited about starting a new diet, it's tempting to jump right in, but your body will thank you if you ease it into the ketogenic diet slowly. Doing so will lessen the severity of any of the "keto flu" symptoms you might experience and make the transition a little easier. Give yourself about three to four weeks from the time you commit to following a ketogenic diet to the day you actually start it 100 percent.

Four Weeks to Keto Success

During the first week cut out all sugary beverages. This includes soda, lemonade, sweetened teas, and flavored waters. If you put sugar in your coffee, scale back—use one teaspoon instead of two. After one week of this remove all desserts and sugary snacks from your diet, including candy, cookies, cakes, muffins, chocolates, and ice cream. Get in the habit of not having dessert after dinner. You want to train your body to stop craving sweets, and one way to do this is to cut them out completely, especially while you're transitioning to a ketogenic diet. On your third week cut out starchy carbohydrates such as pasta, pizza, bread, crackers, rolls, and potatoes. At this point you may have already started to lose weight.

When you start week four, you'll be ready to officially start your ketogenic diet. This is when you should start tracking your macronutrients to make sure you're staying within the correct ratios. Limiting carbohydrates is important, but it's not the only goal; make sure you're also eating plenty of fat and moderate amounts of protein.

Stay Hydrated and Replenish Electrolytes

Staying hydrated is always important, but it's especially vital when you're starting a ketogenic diet. It's not only about drinking water; you also want to replenish your electrolytes. When you start a ketogenic diet, you initially lose water, which takes electrolytes such as sodium and potassium with it. Aim to drink the equivalent of at least half your body weight in ounces. This means that, for example, if you're 180 pounds, you'll want to drink at least 90 ounces of water a day.

You can replenish your electrolytes by drinking a cup of homemade bone broth every day, adding salt to your foods, and drinking waters that are enhanced with electrolytes. Just make sure that the enhanced waters are unflavored, as the flavored waters often contain a lot of sugar and other artificial ingredients.

Keep in mind that the soup stocks and broths that you get at the store are a lot different from the bone broth you make at home. To make an electrolyte-rich bone broth get some high-quality soup bones from your local farmer or butcher. Put these bones in a pot and add enough water to just cover them. Add some salt and pepper, and some bay leaves if you prefer, and let the broth simmer for 12 to 24 hours.

Foods to Avoid

When following the ketogenic diet some foods are strictly off-limits, while others fall into a sort of gray area. Regardless of whether foods are "allowed," you still have to make sure that you're staying within your macronutrient ratios. But remember that just because a food is technically allowed doesn't mean you can eat as much of it as you want. As with any diet, moderation is key. Use these recommendations as a guideline, but always make sure that you're staying within your calculated macronutrient ratios.

Quality Matters

Keep in mind that the quality of your food matters, especially when it comes to fat and protein sources. Ideally, you want to choose meats that are organic, grass-fed, and pasture-raised. Eggs should come from your local farmer or from pasture-raised hens whenever possible. Choose grass-fed butter and organic creams, cheese, fruits, and vegetables. Eating conventional foods won't prevent you from entering a ketogenic state, but high-quality foods are better for your body in general. After all, you are what you eat. Do your best to get the highest quality food you can find and/or afford.

Fats and Oils

Fats and oils provide the basis of your ketogenic diet, so you'll want to make sure you're eating plenty of them. The ketogenic diet is not just a fat free-for-all, though. While following a ketogenic diet there are certain fats that are better for you than others, although which ones fall into which category may surprise you. On the ketogenic diet you should eat plenty of saturated fats in the form of meat, poultry, eggs, butter, and coconut; monounsaturated fats, such as olive oil, nuts, nut butters, and avocado; and natural polyunsaturated fats, such as tuna, salmon, and mackerel. Avoid highly processed polyunsaturated fats, such as canola oil, vegetable oil, and soybean oil. Homemade Mayonnaise is also an easy way to add a dose of fat to every meal (see recipe for Homemade Mayonnaise in Chapter 6).

Proteins

Many of the fat sources mentioned previously—meat, poultry, eggs, butter, nuts, nut butters, and fish—are also loaded with protein. These should be your main protein sources when following a ketogenic diet. Bacon and sausage are other sources of protein that also provide a significant dose of fat. When eating protein make sure to stay within your recommended grams for the day, since your body turns excess protein into glucose, which can kick you out of ketosis.

Fruits and Vegetables

When following a ketogenic diet most fruits fall onto the "do not eat" list. Even though the sugars in fruit are natural sugars, they still raise your blood glucose levels significantly and can kick you out of ketosis. There's not a hard rule that fruit isn't allowed on a ketogenic diet, but you do need to limit your intake. When you do eat fruit, choose fruits that are high in fiber and lower in carbohydrates, such as berries, and limit your portions.

Vegetables are extremely important on a ketogenic diet. They provide the vitamins and minerals that you need to stay healthy and help fill you up without contributing a lot of calories to your day. You do have to be choosy about which vegetables you eat, though, since some are loaded with carbohydrates and do not have a place on a ketogenic diet. As a general rule choose dark green or leafy green vegetables, such as spinach, broccoli, cucumbers, green beans, lettuce, and asparagus. Cauliflower and mushrooms are also good choices for a ketogenic diet. Avoid starchy vegetables, including white potatoes, sweet potatoes, yams, and corn.

Dairy

Full-fat dairy products are a staple on the ketogenic diet. Use butter, heavy cream, sour cream, cream cheese, hard cheese, and cottage cheese to help meet your fat needs. Avoid low-fat dairy products and flavored dairy products, such as fruity yogurt. Flavored yogurt is full of sugar; serving for serving, some versions contain as much sugar and carbohydrates as soda!

Beverages

As with any diet plan, when it comes to beverages, water is your best bet. Make sure to drink at least half of your body weight in ounces. Coffee and tea are also permitted on a ketogenic diet, but they must be unsweetened or sweetened with an approved sweetener, such as stevia or erythritol. Avoid sodas, flavored waters, sweetened teas, sweetened lemonade, and fruit juices. You can infuse plain water with fresh herbs, such as mint or basil, to give yourself a little variety.

Although artificially sweetened beverages are allowed on a ketogenic diet because they don't contain any carbohydrates, try to avoid them. Some research shows that even though artificial sweeteners don't contain any calories, they can contribute to weight gain. Plus, part of the goal is to try to get rid of your sweet tooth, and drinking sweetened beverages won't help you do that.

Embracing the Fat Bomb

Fat bombs are low-carbohydrate, high-fat recipes or foods that include a high percentage of fat and a low percentage of carbohydrates. Fat bombs were originally created as pure fat snacks to reach your fat macronutrient goal for the day when following a ketogenic diet. Since the ketogenic diet requires such high levels of fat for the body to enter and stay in ketosis, fat bombs are an easy solution to help dieters reach their fat requirements each day. Over time and with the widespread use of the diet the concept of the fat bomb has widened a little to include small meals with an adequate ratio of protein to fat that also keep the carbohydrate content to a minimum. These snacks and meals, when consumed throughout the day, will help you successfully maintain your macronutrient ratios for the diet while providing necessary nutrients and keeping you satisfied.

Using Fat Bombs for Success on the Ketogenic Diet

Fat bombs can be used to balance your macronutrient intake of fat and protein while leaving your carbohydrate intake adequately low. You can start your day with a savory, egg-based fat bomb for breakfast to get a head start in consuming healthy fats and to make sure your blood sugar will be stable for the rest of the day. Or, you can add in a fat-bomb snack in the middle of your day to combat that midafternoon slump and problematic sugar craving. Another idea is to use a small fat-bomb dinner to keep your caloric intake as low as needed and to fill your need for fat. These are just some of the ways a fat bomb can be your invaluable ally for your success with a ketogenic diet.

Enjoying Liquid Fat Bombs

Convenience will make it easier to successfully stick to your eating plan. Liquid fat bombs are a great way to help you get the right balance of fats, proteins, and carbohydrates for your body. When pressed for time it can be invaluable to be able to throw a few ingredients into a blender and make it a meal. Liquid fat bombs can be easily created, easily transported, and easily shared. They will provide the right macronutrients your body needs, some essential nutrients, and a lot of great flavor to your diet.

Using Savory Fat Bombs

Many fat-bomb recipes feature sweet ingredients to make the fats more palatable. However, as you adjust to adding fat bombs to your diet, you'll need to balance savory with sweet. In addition to the benefits of savory fat bombs as meal replacers there is another very important reason to use savory instead of just eating the sweet, "treat-like" ones. Sugar consumption is directly related to insulin release into the bloodstream. Your body becomes so trained to expect a blood sugar spike following the ingestion of sweet-flavored foods that it creates an almost automatic response. It is clinically proven that the ingestion of noncaloric sweeteners will still trigger an insulin response in the body, especially if you are insulin resistant. That mechanism is proven by the fact that a sweet-flavored treat with the same macronutrient ratios as a savory one will make you hungry much sooner. When weaning yourself from the habit of sugar the sweet flavor alone can become a trigger for powerful cravings, even if the sweetener had zero carbohydrates in it.

Adapting to a High-Fat Diet

The concept of a "fat bomb" can be quite shocking if you are not familiar with the principles and challenges of a ketogenic diet. At first a fat bomb may sound quite unappealing to you, but once you understand its value and application within the diet, you will be eager to try all the enticing and flavorful ways to get more fat into your body.

One of the hardest parts of the ketogenic diet is matching your required fat intake, especially at the beginning. If you are transitioning from a long-term, low-fat dieting plan, chances are you forgot how to use fats in your diet.

Current low-fat recipe trends combined with ready-made "healthy" meals sold in supermarkets will not help you meet your weight-loss or health goals. Often, they are high in carbohydrates and sugar, despite being labeled as "healthy" because they are low in fat. Once you start keeping track of your macros on a ketogenic diet, you'll find yourself reaching your carbohydrate limit early in the day, while you still have a lot of calories left to fill in the form of fat and protein. The fat bomb is the easy solution for this seemingly impossible problem.

Calculating Your Macronutrient Ratio

The first thing you need to do to calculate your macronutrient ratio is to figure out how many calories you should be eating. There are several online calculators that can calculate this number for you, but to do it yourself you can use a method called the Mifflin-St Jeor formula, which looks like this:

Men: 10 × weight (kg) + 6.25 × height (cm) − 5 × age (y) + 5
Women: 10 × weight (kg) + 6.25 × height (cm) − 5 × age (y) − 161

To make this explanation easier let's try using the equation with a thirty-year-old, 160-pound (72.7 kg) woman who is 5 feet 5 inches (165.1 cm) tall. When you plug this woman's statistics into the Mifflin-St Jeor formula, you can see that she should be eating 1,448 calories per day. Now you'll use the estimated macronutrient percentages to calculate how much of each nutrient she needs to consume in order to follow a successful ketogenic diet plan.

Years ago, unless you had the fancy, expensive software that nutritionists use, the only way to track your macronutrients was by looking up each food item, writing down its carbohydrate, protein, and fat content, and adding it all up. Nowadays, there are several apps that you can download on your phone that will do the work for you. Make your life easier by downloading one of these apps—a popular one is MyFitnessPal—and tracking everything you eat.

Macro Number for Carbohydrates

On a ketogenic diet, carbohydrates should provide only 5 to 10 percent of the calories you consume. Many ketogenic dieters stay at the low end of 5 percent, but the exact amount you need depends on your body. Unfortunately, there is no one-size-fits-all approach to this, so you'll have to do a little trial and error. You can pick a percentage that feels right for you and try that out for a couple of weeks. If you don't see the results you want, you'll have to adjust your nutrient ratios and calculate them again. Getting 7 percent of your calories from carbohydrates is a good place to start.

To calculate how many grams of carbohydrates this is, multiply 7 percent by the total number of calories, which in the earlier example is 1,448, and then divide by 4 (since carbohydrates contain 4 calories per gram). The number you're left with is the amount of carbohydrates in grams you should eat per day. In this example the number is 25 grams.

Total Carbohydrates versus Net Carbohydrates

When counting carbohydrates on a ketogenic diet plan, you want to pay attention to net carbohydrates, not total carbohydrates. Net carbohydrates are the amount of carbohydrates left over after you subtract grams of fiber from total grams of carbohydrates. If a particular food contains 10 grams of carbohydrates, but 7 grams come from fiber, the total number of net carbohydrates is 3 grams. You count the 3 grams toward your daily total, rather than the 10 grams.

Macro Number for Fat

After you've calculated carbohydrates, move on to fat. Again, the exact amount you'll need depends on you as an individual, but consuming 75 percent of your calories from fat is a good place to start. To figure out the amount of fat you need in grams multiply the number of calories you need (in this example, 1,448) by 75 percent and then divide by 9 (since fat contains 9 calories per gram). The number you're left with is the total grams of fat you need for the day. In this example it's 121 grams.

Macro Number for Protein

Once you've calculated carbohydrates and fat, protein is easy. The remainder of your calories, which equates to 18 percent, should come from protein. To figure out this number in grams multiply the total number of calories by 18 percent and then divide by 4 (since protein contains 4 calories per gram). The number you're left with is the total grams of protein you need for the day. In this example it's 65 grams.

Recalculating Macronutrients

As your body changes, your macronutrient ranges may also change. When following a ketogenic diet it's beneficial to recalculate your nutrient needs regularly—about once per month. If your needs change, adjust your diet accordingly.

Planning Meals for Long-Term Success

Planning your meals is vital to your long-term success on a ketogenic diet. There is a popular quote, most often credited to Benjamin Franklin, that goes something like this: "When you fail to plan, you plan to fail." It's true. The best way to ensure success is to plan your weekly meals, prepare meals in advance, and always make sure you have ketogenic-approved snacks on hand.

Meal Planning

Take one night a week and write out everything you will eat all week. Plan your meals and your snacks and then compile a grocery list for what you'll need in order to execute these meals and snacks. You may choose to make your meal planning day your shopping day as well. Get everything you need in one swoop and then don't stray from your plan.

Meal Prep

Once you know what you're going to eat all week, you may decide that you want to cook each meal individually, or you may decide that spending a few hours prepping your meals makes more sense for you. If you choose the latter, pick a day when you don't have any other commitments and spend a few hours in the kitchen preparing your meals for the entire week. You can make a quiche, a couple of ketogenic-friendly casseroles, and a big pot of soup. Divide each meal into to-go containers and store them in the refrigerator so that they're ready to go when you are.

Say Goodbye to Convenience Foods

When you're on a specialized diet such as the ketogenic one, there is really no such thing as convenience foods. You have to be prepared at all times. You might have to take meals and snacks with you everywhere you go, but it's a small price to pay for the way you'll feel. Pack a lunch every day and keep nonperishable snacks, like fat bombs, coconut shavings, nuts, and seeds in your car, in your desk at work, and in your purse or briefcase.

Don't Make It Complicated

It's tempting to want to create elaborate meal plans that feature a new gourmet entrée each night, but for most people that's just not realistic. You have to make sure that your new diet plan can fit into your lifestyle; otherwise, you won't be able to stick to it. Keep things simple by eating the same thing for breakfast three times a week and using leftovers from dinner for the next day's lunch. You can double or triple recipes to prepare meals in bulk and then freeze them for another day when you don't have the time to cook.

Starting a new diet is not easy; it takes dedication and preparation. You'll have to do some fine-tuning and rearranging to figure out what works for you, but once you get the hang of it, it will become second nature.

2

Understanding Ketosis

Your body is highly intelligent. It knows exactly what it wants and what it needs to do to get what it wants, and the main thing it wants is energy. Without energy your cells would starve, and you would die. In order to make sure that it always has access to energy, your body has several metabolic pathways it can use to convert the food you eat into usable energy. The default metabolic pathway is one that uses the glucose from carbohydrates as fuel. As long as you provide your body with carbohydrates, it will use them as energy, storing fat in the process. When you deny your body carbohydrates, it has to turn somewhere else to get the energy it needs to live.

What Is Ketosis?

Your body's second preferred source of energy is fat; when carbohydrates are not easily accessible, your body turns to fat to get the energy it needs. When this happens the liver breaks down fat into fatty acids and then breaks down these fatty acids into an energy-rich substance called ketones or ketone bodies. The presence of ketone bodies in the blood is called ketosis. The goal of a ketogenic diet is to kick your body into long-term ketosis, essentially turning it into a fat-burning machine.

How Your Body Obtains Energy

Your cells need a constant supply of energy to stay alive and keep you alive. Even when you're sitting on the couch doing nothing, your body is generating energy for your cells. Since energy cannot be created, only converted from one form to another, your body needs to get this energy from somewhere, so it uses the food you eat. Your body can use each macronutrient—carbohydrates, fat, and protein—for energy. The biochemical process of obtaining energy is a complicated one, but it's important to understand the basics so you can get a feel for how ketosis works on a cellular level.

Energy from Protein

Protein is the body's least favorite macronutrient to use as energy. This is because protein serves so many other functions in the body, way more than any other macronutrient. Protein provides structural support to every cell in your body and helps maintain your body tissues. Proteins act as enzymes that play a role in all of the chemical reactions in your body. Without these enzymes these chemical reactions would be so slow that your body wouldn't be able to carry out basic processes like digestion and metabolism, and you wouldn't be able to survive. Proteins also help maintain fluid and acid-base balance, help transport substances such as oxygen through the body and waste out of the body, and act as antibodies to keep your immune system strong and help fight off illness.

Proteins are made up of amino acids. When you eat proteins, your body breaks them down into their individual amino acids, which are then converted into sugars through a process called deamination. Your body can use these protein-turned-sugars as a form of energy, but that means your body isn't using the amino acids for those other important functions. It's best to avoid forcing the body to use protein for energy, and you do that by providing it with the other nutrients it needs. That being said, if the body has no other choice but to use protein for energy, it will.

Protein Breakdown

This process of using protein for energy is what makes extreme calorie restriction dangerous. If you are on a diet that doesn't provide enough calories, your body begins to break down the protein in your muscles for energy, which can lead to muscle loss or muscle wasting in addition to nutritional deficiencies.

Energy from Carbohydrates

Although your body is adept at using any food that's available for energy, it always turns to carbohydrates first. When you eat carbohydrates, they are broken down into glucose or another sugar that's easily converted to glucose. Glucose is absorbed through the walls of the small intestine and then enters your body by way of your bloodstream, which causes your blood glucose levels to rise. As soon as the glucose enters your blood, your pancreas sends out insulin to pick up the sugar and carry it to your cells so they can use it as energy.

Once your cells have used all the glucose they need at that time, much of the remaining glucose is converted into glycogen (the storage form of glucose), which is then stored in the liver and muscles. The liver has a limited ability to store glycogen, though; it can only store enough glycogen to provide you with energy for about 24 hours. All the extra glucose that can't be stored is converted into triglycerides, the storage form of fat, and stored in your fat cells.

When you don't eat for a few hours and your blood sugar starts to drop, your body will call on the glycogen stored in the liver and muscles for energy before anything else. The pancreas releases a hormone called glucagon, which triggers the release of glucose from the glycogen stored in your liver to help raise your blood sugar levels. This process is called glycogenolysis. The glycogen stored in your liver is used exclusively to increase your blood glucose levels, while the glycogen stored in your muscles is used strictly as fuel for your muscles. When you eat carbohydrates again, your body uses the glucose it gets from them to replenish those glycogen stores. If you regularly eat carbohydrates, your body never has a problem getting access to glucose for energy, and the stored fat stays where it is—in your fat cells.

Energy from Fat

The body prefers to use carbohydrates for energy because they're easily accessible and fast-acting, but in the absence of carbohydrates your body turns to fat. The fat from the food you eat is broken down into fatty acids, which enter the bloodstream through the walls of the small intestine. Most of your cells can directly use fatty acids for energy, but some specialized cells, such as the cells in your brain and your muscles, can't run on fatty acids directly. To appease these cells and give them the energy they need your body uses fatty acids to make ketones.

The Creation of Ketones

When your body doesn't have access to glucose—for example, during times of fasting or when intentionally following a low-carbohydrate diet—it turns to fat for energy. Fat is taken to the liver, where it is broken down into glycerol and fatty acids through a process called beta-oxidation. The fatty acid molecules are further broken down through a process called ketogenesis, and a specific ketone body called acetoacetate is formed.

Over time as your body becomes adapted to using ketones as fuel, your muscles convert acetoacetate into beta-hydroxybutyrate (BHB), which is the preferred ketogenic source of energy for your brain, and acetone, most of which is expelled from the body as waste.

The glycerol created during beta-oxidation goes through a process called gluconeogenesis. During gluconeogenesis the body converts glycerol into glucose that your body can use for energy. Your body can also convert excess protein into glucose. Your body does need some glucose to function, but it doesn't need carbohydrates to get it. It does a good job of converting whatever it can into the simple sugar.

Ketosis and Weight Loss

Now that you understand how your body creates energy and how ketones are formed, you may be left wondering how this translates into weight loss. When you eat a lot of carbohydrates, your body happily burns them for energy and stores any excess as glycogen in your liver or as triglycerides in your fat cells. When you take carbohydrates out of the equation, your body depletes its glycogen stores in the liver and muscles and then turns to fat for energy. Your body obtains energy from the fat in the food you eat, but it also uses the triglycerides, or fats, stored in your fat cells. When your body starts burning stored fat, your fat cells shrink, and you begin to lose weight and become leaner.

Triglycerides are the storage form of fat in your body and the food you eat. When you eat more food than your body needs for energy, it is converted into triglycerides and stored in your fat cells for later use.

Keto-Adaptation

During the first few weeks on the ketogenic diet your body undergoes a series of changes to adapt its functions for burning fat as the preferred fuel source. This process is called keto-adaptation. Some of these adaptations include adapting the brain to burn ketones instead of glucose. The brain will be able to use a maximum of 75 percent ketones for energy; the rest will always have to be glucose. As stated, the body will be able to produce its own glucose from protein and triglycerides.

How to Induce Ketosis

Inducing ketosis is not an easy task, but once you get the hang of it, it can become second nature. The first step in inducing ketosis is to severely limit carbohydrate consumption, but that's not enough. You must limit your protein consumption as well. Traditional low-carbohydrate diets don't induce ketosis because they allow a high intake of protein. Because your body is able to convert excess protein into glucose, your body never switches over to burning fat as fuel. You can induce ketosis by following a high-fat diet that allows moderate amounts of protein and allows only a small amount of carbohydrates—or what is called a ketogenic diet.

The exact percentage of each macronutrient you need to kick your body into ketosis may vary from person to person, but in general the macronutrient ratio falls into the following ranges:

- 60–75 percent of calories from fat
- 15–30 percent of calories from protein
- 5–10 percent of calories from carbohydrates

This largely differs from both a standard low-carbohydrate diet, which typically allows more calories to come from protein, and the traditional dietary reference intakes set by the National Academy of Medicine.

Currently, the National Academy of Medicine recommends getting 45–65 percent of your calories from carbohydrates, 20–35 percent of your calories from fat, and 10–35 percent of your calories from protein. Although the individual recommendations of low-carbohydrate diets differ based on which one you follow, they typically allow about 20 percent of calories from carbohydrates, 25–30 percent from protein, and 55–65 percent from fat.

Once you're in ketosis, you have to continue with the high-fat, low-carbohydrate, moderate-protein plan. Eating too many carbohydrates or too much protein can kick you out of ketosis at any time by providing your body with enough glucose to stop using fat as fuel.

Signs That You Are in Ketosis

Signs that you're in ketosis may start appearing after only one week of following a true ketogenic diet. For some people it can take longer—as much as three months. The amount of time it takes for you to start seeing signs that your body is burning fat for fuel largely depends on you as an individual. When signs do start to show, they are pretty similar across the board.

Keto "Flu"

"Keto flu" or "low-carb flu" commonly affects people in the first few days of starting a ketogenic diet. Of course the ketogenic diet doesn't actually cause the flu, but the phenomenon is given the term because its symptoms closely resemble that of the flu. It would be more accurate to refer to this stage as a carbohydrate withdrawal because that's really what it is. When you take carbohydrates away, it causes altered hormonal states and electrolyte imbalances that are responsible for the associated symptoms. The basic symptoms include headache, nausea, upset stomach, sleepiness, fatigue, abdominal cramps, diarrhea, and lack of mental clarity, or what is commonly referred to as "brain fog."

The duration of symptoms varies—it depends on you as an individual, but typically a "keto flu" lasts anywhere from a couple of days to a week. In rare cases it can last up to two weeks. Some of the symptoms of the "keto flu" are associated with dehydration, because in the beginning stages of ketosis you lose a lot of water weight. With that lost fluid you also lose electrolytes. You can replenish these electrolytes by drinking enhanced waters (but make sure they are not sweetened) and drinking lots of homemade bone broth. This may help lessen the severity of the symptoms.

Bad Breath

Unfortunately, bad breath is another early sign that you're in ketosis. When you're in ketosis, your body creates acetone as a waste product. Some of this acetone is released in your breath, giving it a fruity or ammonia-like quality. You can combat bad breath by chewing on fresh mint leaves and drinking plenty of water, since bad breath is also associated with dehydration.

Decreased Appetite and Nausea

As your body adapts to a ketogenic diet, you may have a decreased appetite. This is because you're providing your body with plenty of fat and protein, which are both highly satiating, and not a lot of carbohydrates. Nausea associated with "keto flu" can also decrease your appetite. When you reach this stage, it's important that you eat even if you feel like you aren't hungry. You want to make sure your body is getting enough calories and nutrients, especially in this time of transition.

Increased Energy and Mental Clarity

When the fog begins to clear and your body starts to become keto-adapted, the uncomfortable symptoms you were feeling will dissipate, and you'll begin to see the benefits of following a ketogenic diet. One of the first beneficial signs many people experience is an increase in energy. When your body breaks down fat instead of carbohydrates, more energy is produced gram for gram, leaving you feeling alert and energized.

Many mental issues, such as brain fog and problems with memory, are caused by what is called neurotoxicity, the exposure of the nervous system to toxic substances. For the brain, exposure to too much glucose can result in neurotoxicity. When you reduce the supply of glucose in your body, and your brain starts to use ketones as fuel, the toxicity levels diminish. As a result you may be able to think more clearly, focus better, and have better memory recall.

Other possible signs of ketosis include:

- Cold hands and feet
- Increased urinary frequency
- Difficulty sleeping
- Metallic taste in the mouth
- Dry mouth
- Increased thirst

Measurable Ketones

Your body is pretty good at letting you know when you're in ketosis without any testing, but if you desire you can test your ketone levels with urine strips or a blood meter. Urine strips allow you to easily test for the presence of ketones in your urine, while blood meters can test for ketones with a small blood sample from a prick in your finger. These testing methods tend to be more reliable than just trusting the presence of symptoms, and if you really want to know if you're producing ketones, they're a great way to find out, but sometimes they can be inaccurate.

Although these signs are common among many people who follow a ketogenic diet, your experience may be different. Every body is unique, so it's impossible to say exactly what your personal experience will be. Keep in mind that in the early stages of ketosis your symptoms may be unpleasant, but as your body adapts, you will begin to experience the benefits of following a ketogenic diet plan.

Managing Keto Symptoms

The initial symptoms of a ketogenic diet are uncomfortable, but if you choose to ride it out, you can rest assured that in time they will go away. If the thought of being uncomfortable is really too much to bear, there are a few things you can try to help decrease the chances of experiencing symptoms or at least lessen their severity.

Like anything else, symptoms tend to be the worst when you transition to a ketogenic diet cold turkey. If you've been following a high-carbohydrate, low-fat diet for years—even decades—abruptly asking your body to run on fat instead is like a slap in the face. Instead of jumping right into a ketogenic diet, transition slowly.

Start by gradually eliminating non-nutritive carbohydrate sources, such as soda, desserts, sugary snacks, pasta, and pizza, over a period of a few weeks. As you eliminate these carbohydrate sources, increase the amount of fats you eat—coconut, avocado, and cheese, for example. When you've gotten used to the general principles of the diet, start tracking specific numbers and macronutrient ratios.

Snack Regularly and Drink Water

Eating a high-fat, moderate-protein snack, such as a fat bomb—a snack that serves as a concentrated source of healthy fats—may help ease certain symptoms, including headache and irritability. When you're first starting a ketogenic diet, make sure to snack regularly to keep yourself from getting too hungry. You may also consider protein shakes with amino acid supplements, which can help soften the transition. Just make sure these shakes are low in carbohydrates and don't contain a bevy of artificial ingredients.

Drink Water

Many of the symptoms, such as bad breath, are associated with being dehydrated. Drink plenty of water while you're transitioning and for the entire duration of your ketogenic diet. In addition to keeping you hydrated water dilutes the ketone bodies, which can help alleviate symptoms.

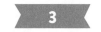

Fat Is Your Friend

If you're one of the people who followed a low-fat diet and failed to lose weight or failed to see any other major health improvements, don't worry; you're in the company of millions. When the popularity of the low-fat diet surged, many followers found themselves gaining more weight. Removing fat from your diet was supposed to make you thinner and healthier, but it did just the opposite. When people started replacing fats with carbohydrates and low-fat alternatives, the incidences of diabetes and obesity began to skyrocket. Could the beloved low-fat diet be to blame? Absolutely.

The Skinny of the Keto Diet

The ketogenic diet is not a new trend or a fad. The high-fat, low-carbohydrate diet has been around since the 1920s when it was used for nearly two decades as the main treatment method for difficult-to-control epilepsy in young children. Although the diet worked remarkably well, eventually it fell by the wayside when antiseizure medications became more readily available.

Fat Can Make You Healthy

Like anything, if you overdo it, too much fat can cause weight gain, but it's not the scary monster it's been made out to be. In fact it's the opposite. Dietary fat is an absolute necessity. Eating fat can help you lose weight and build muscle; it also increases mental clarity, gives you energy, improves mood, contributes to glowing skin and better eye health, boosts your immune system, and leads to better brain function. And here's a big shocker: fat has been shown to improve cholesterol ratio and reduce heart disease risk. That's right: eating fat is actually linked with a healthier heart and lower cholesterol levels! While fat has a bad reputation, it's carbohydrates and processed vegetable oils, like canola, corn, and soybean, that are largely responsible for weight gain and the increasing rates of chronic health conditions, like heart disease, diabetes, and autoimmune disorders. Limiting carbohydrates and sugars and replacing them with both saturated and unsaturated fats—the basis of the ketogenic diet—can help you lose weight today as well as keep you healthy for years to come.

Low-Fat Diet Myths

Fat is not your enemy; sugar is. And that applies to all forms of sugar, not only the granulated stuff that you put in your coffee in the morning. Sure, the sugar in fruit is packaged with vitamin C, potassium, fiber, and other valuable nutrients, which makes it a far superior choice over regular old sugar, but overdoing it can actually hinder weight-loss efforts and set you up for other health problems. But before delving too deeply into sugar it's important to spend some time debunking the myths that have surrounded the word *fat* for years.

As the low-fat diet began to gain popularity, there was also an increase in the availability of low-fat food items, such as cookies and candy bars. To create these items manufacturers removed fat and replaced it with sugar to keep it palatable so consumers would continue to buy the product. These packaged food items were lower in fat, but they were higher in sugar and contained the same, if not more, calories.

Carbohydrate Addiction

Carbohydrate addiction is a real thing. Some research shows that carbohydrates activate certain stimuli in the brain that can be dependence forming. Carbohydrate addicts have uncontrollable cravings, and when they do eat, they tend to binge. In a carbohydrate addict the removal of carbohydrates can cause withdrawal symptoms, such as dizziness and irritability, and intense cravings.

Eating Fat Does Not Make You Fat

On the surface the theory that eating fat makes you fat seems like a no-brainer. Of the three macronutrients—protein, carbohydrates, and fat—fat contains the most calories per gram. Protein and carbohydrates have 4 calories per gram, while fat contains more than twice that at 9 calories per gram. It would make sense that if you cut out fat or replace fat with protein or carbohydrates at each meal, you would be saving yourself a ton of calories throughout the course of the day. While technically you would save on calories, it doesn't lead to sustainable weight loss.

Why We Gain Weight

In order to understand why fat doesn't make you fat you have to understand how you gain weight in the first place. The simple explanation is this: You start thinking about food, and your body secretes insulin in response. The insulin triggers a response that tells your body to store fatty acids instead of using them for energy, so you get hungry. When you get hungry, you eat. If you're on a low-fat diet, your lunch may consist of two slices of whole-wheat toast with a couple of slices of turkey—no cheese, no mayo—and an apple on the side. If you've subscribed to the low-fat diet theory, this seems like a healthy meal, but in reality it's loaded with carbohydrates that pass through your digestive system quickly, causing significant spikes in blood sugar, and it has virtually no fat.

Don't Overdo It

Your body quickly breaks down your high-carbohydrate meal, which sends a rush of glucose into your bloodstream. Your body responds to this glucose by secreting more insulin, which carries the glucose out of your blood and into your cells. Once the glucose levels drop, you get hungry again, your body secretes more insulin, and the cycle starts over.

Now here's where you'll want to pay close attention. Your body's main regulator of fat metabolism is insulin. Insulin controls lipoprotein lipase, or LPL, an enzyme that pulls fat into your cells. The higher your insulin levels, the more fat LPL pulls into your cells. Translation: When insulin levels increase, you store fat. When insulin levels drop, you burn fat for energy. The main thing that affects insulin levels is carbohydrates, not fat. So, when you eat a lot of carbohydrates, your insulin levels increase, which increases your LPL levels, which increases your storage of fat.

It's important to remember that overdoing it on any of the nutrients will lead to weight gain. Regularly exceeding your calorie needs will cause weight gain, regardless of whether you do it with carbohydrates, protein, or fat—but fat is not the major culprit when it comes to weight gain.

The truth is, carbohydrates are a fast-acting source of energy for your body, but they don't do a lot to fill you up. Even carbohydrates that are loaded with fiber are far less satiating than either protein or fat. If you want your meal to be truly satisfying, make sure it contains plenty of fat.

Myth: Cholesterol Causes Heart Disease

The cholesterol you eat actually has very little impact on your blood cholesterol levels for two reasons. The first reason is that your body doesn't absorb dietary cholesterol very efficiently. Most of the cholesterol you eat goes right through your digestive tract and never even enters your bloodstream. The second reason is that the amount of cholesterol in your blood is tightly controlled by your body. When you eat a lot of dietary cholesterol, your body shuts down its own production of cholesterol to compensate. There is a percentage of the population, however, that is hypersensitive to dietary cholesterol. For these people—about 25 percent of the population—dietary cholesterol does cause modest increases in both LDL (low-density lipoprotein) and HDL (high-density lipoprotein) levels, but even so, the increased cholesterol levels do not increase the risk of heart disease. In fact both the Framingham Heart Study and the Kuakini Honolulu Heart Program/Kuakini Honolulu-Asia Aging Study found the opposite to be true: low cholesterol levels were actually associated with increased risk of death. A separate study published in the *Journal of the American Medical Association* reported findings that neither high LDL ("bad" cholesterol) levels nor low HDL ("good" cholesterol) levels were important risk factors for death from coronary artery disease or heart attack.

Importance of Cholesterol

Cholesterol is absolutely essential for your survival. This lipoprotein, as it is physiologically classified, performs three major functions. It makes up the bile acids that help you digest food; it allows the body to make vitamin D and other essential hormones such as estrogen and testosterone; and it is a component of the outer coating of every one of your cells. Without cholesterol your body would literally crumble.

Most of the cholesterol in your blood (75 percent) is actually made in your body. Only 25 percent comes from the food you eat. If you followed a completely cholesterol-free diet, your body would compensate by increasing its cholesterol production by the liver to keep your blood levels steady. That's because your body needs cholesterol to survive. Without sufficient cholesterol your immune system cannot properly function, you cannot produce sufficient steroid hormones (leading to severe sex hormone imbalances), your cell membranes get weak, and you end up with impaired memory and brain function.

Moderation Is Key

Now that's not to say that you should throw all caution to the wind when it comes to cholesterol, but you need to pay attention to the right thing, and that's the size of the cholesterol particles in your bloodstream rather than the total numbers. Cholesterol comes in two forms: large particles that "bounce" off the arterial walls and small, dense particles that stick to the walls of your arteries and contribute to arterial blockage, which can eventually lead to heart disease. The problem is that so much focus is placed on the total numbers that many people fail to pay attention to cholesterol particle size.

According to Dr. Mark Hyman, a functional medicine doctor at the UltraWellness Center in Lenox, Massachusetts, it's not fat that causes the accumulation of small, dense cholesterol particles in your blood, it's sugar. And that's sugar in any form, including refined carbohydrates. Sugar decreases the amount of the large cholesterol particles in your blood, creates the small damaging cholesterol particles, increases triglyceride levels, and contributes to prediabetes.

Can Saturated Fat Cause Heart Disease?

The other widespread belief is that eating saturated fat causes an increase in the amount of cholesterol in your blood, which in turn causes heart disease or increases your risk of heart disease. This theory was developed from some human and animal studies that were done decades ago. However, more recent research calls these theories into question.

In 2010 the *American Journal of Clinical Nutrition* did a meta-analysis of several studies that investigated the relationship between saturated fat and heart disease and concluded that there is no significant evidence to make the claim that dietary saturated fat is associated with increased risk of coronary heart disease or cardio-vascular disease, in general. In fact several of the studies the journal investigated showed a positive inverse relationship, which means that a higher intake of saturated fat was actually associated with a lower incidence of heart disease.

Researchers went even further to suggest that more analysis be done to deter-mine whether the nutrients that replaced saturated fat actually had more of an influ-ence on the risk of developing heart disease. After all, the nutrient that was used to replace saturated fat on low-fat diets was carbohydrates.

Why Fat Is Your Friend

Fat is an integral part of every cell in your body. This macronutrient is a major component of your cell membranes, which hold each cell together. Every single cell in your body, from the cells in your brain to the cells in your heart to the cells in your lungs, is dependent on fat for survival. Fat is especially important for your brain, which is made up of 60 percent fat and cholesterol.

Fat and cholesterol are used as building blocks for many hormones, which help regulate metabolism, control growth and development, and maintain bone and muscle mass, among many other things. Fat is vital for proper immune function, helps regulate body temperature, and serves as a source of protection for your major organs. Fat surrounds all of your vital organs to provide a sort of cushion for protection against falls and trauma. Fat also helps boost metabolic function and plays a role in keeping you lean.

Fat is an essential nutrient. This means that you need to ingest it through the foods you eat because the body cannot make what it needs on its own. Fat is composed of individual molecules called fatty acids. Two of these fatty acids, omega-3 fatty acids and omega-6 fatty acids, are absolutely essential for good health. Omega-3 fatty acids play a crucial role in brain function and growth and development, while omega-6 fatty acids help regulate metabolism and maintain bone health. Fat also allows you to absorb and digest other essential nutrients, such as vitamins A, D, E, and K and beta-carotene. Without enough fat in your diet you wouldn't be able to absorb any of these nutrients, and you would eventually develop nutritional deficiencies.

As if that weren't enough, fat is a major source of energy for your body. The fact that each gram of fat contains 9 calories is actually a good thing. This makes it a compact source of energy that your body can use easily and efficiently. Unlike with carbohydrates, which your body can store only in limited amounts, your body has an unlimited ability to store fat for later use. When food intake falls short, as between meals or while you're sleeping, your body calls on its fat reservoirs for energy. This physiological process is what the entire ketogenic diet is based on.

Burn Away Your Glucose First

Your body needs a continuous source of energy to maintain its functions. The body's preferred source of energy, because it's fast-acting and easily accessible, is glucose, which comes from carbohydrates. When you give your body access to glucose, it stores fat in your fat cells for later use. When you deprive the body of glucose, it turns to fat for energy.

Endurance athletes use the terms "hitting a wall" or "bonking" to describe the point at which they've depleted their glycogen stores and no longer have access to a quick form of energy. Bonking usually manifests as sudden fatigue or a complete loss of energy. When you see marathon runners drinking glucose shots during a race, it's because they want to replenish glycogen stores quickly so that they have enough energy to finish.

Reducing Body Fat

Now that you know what causes your body to store fat, the obvious next question is, "How do you use that knowledge to help reduce your body fat?" The quick answer, and one that may seem counterintuitive at this point, is to eat more fat, but it's not that simple. You can't simply add fat to a diet that's full of carbohydrates and loaded with protein and expect the weight to fall off. You have to make a strategic plan to follow a diet that allows you to eat a significant amount of fat while also limiting carbohydrate intake and eating a moderate amount of protein. In other words: a ketogenic diet.

The Truth about Fat Cells

Researchers at the Karolinska Institutet in Stockholm, Sweden, found that the number of fat cells you have as an adult remains the same no matter how much weight you lose. When you lose weight, the number of fat cells doesn't actually decrease; the cells just shrink in size, essentially taking up less room and making you look leaner.

The Importance of a Healthy Body Fat Level

Fat is important, there's no doubt about that, but too much on your body can be bad for your health. Having excess body fat increases your risk of various health problems, including:

- Type 2 diabetes
- Heart disease
- Gallstones
- Sleep apnea
- Certain types of cancers
- High blood pressure
- Stroke
- Osteoarthritis
- Fatty liver disease
- Infertility
- Kidney disease
- Gestational diabetes

Reducing the amount of fat you carry on your body can help reduce your risk of developing these chronic conditions, even if you have a family history of them.

Feeling Satisfied While Losing Weight

One of the biggest complaints you'll hear from dieters on a weight-loss program is that they don't feel satisfied. They're always hungry, or the food just isn't good. This is where most diets fail. If you're always hungry on a diet, what are the chances that you're going to be able to stick to it long term? Probably close to zero. No one wants to be hungry all the time. Also, consistently eating foods that lack any flavor and always leave you wanting more is a recipe for disaster. At some point your cravings for delicious, satiating foods are going to triumph over your determination to lose weight, and you're going to give in to temptation—and probably in a big way. Feelings of deprivation are one of the biggest causes of eventual binges. When you binge, you gain weight. So, the key to a lasting weight-loss diet plan is to fight off hunger as best you can. This is where fat shines.

Of the three macronutrients, fat is the most satiating. Sure, it's the calorie-densest, too, but it helps you fill up faster and keeps you full longer, which means that you're likely to take in fewer calories over the long term, and you're less prone to uncontrollable binges. When you cut fat out of your diet, it's hard to reach that point when you really feel satisfied. This is why people on low-fat diets complain of being hungry all the time. Fat also adds a ton of flavor to food, so when you eat fat you're actually enjoying the food you're eating, which makes you more likely to stick to your diet plan. Sounds like a no-brainer, right?

Foods with a high fat content tend to taste so good because many different flavors dissolve in fats. Butter especially works as an excellent carrier for a wide variety of flavors, including spices, vanilla, and other fat-soluble ingredients. The human body is also genetically programmed to seek out high-energy foods. Because of this, fatty foods are inherently perceived as more flavorful.

4

Benefits, Risks, and Concerns of the Keto Diet

When you mention the term "ketogenic diet" to someone, you'll usually get one of two responses. The first will be something along the lines of, "Oh, I've heard of that. Tell me more." The second will be more like, "Oh, I've heard of that. It might be really dangerous. Be careful." While there are some individuals who should not follow a ketogenic diet, many others can significantly benefit from one. Confusion over the words *ketosis* and *ketoacidosis* is one of the major reasons people are quick to say that a ketogenic diet is dangerous.

Ketosis versus Ketoacidosis

When discussing a ketogenic diet it's important to differentiate between the terms ketosis and ketoacidosis. A properly planned ketogenic diet is perfectly safe, while ketoacidosis is a dangerous metabolic state that mostly affects type 1 diabetics or those with impaired insulin production.

The levels of ketones associated with ketoacidosis are about three to five times higher than the levels associated with nutritional ketosis. As long as your ketone levels stay in a nutritional ketosis range, you're not at risk for ketoacidosis.

Ketosis is regulated by insulin. Insulin controls the creation of ketone bodies and regulates the flow of fatty acids into the blood. In a healthy individual ketosis is tightly controlled; insulin does not allow ketone bodies to reach toxic levels. Because type 1 diabetics do not produce adequate amounts of insulin, their bodies are unable to regulate ketones in the same way. As a result ketones can accumulate in the blood, turning it into an acidic and potentially dangerous environment. When this happens it can lead to ketoacidosis, a dangerous metabolic state in which excessive amounts of ketones are produced.

The Basics of Type 1 Diabetes

Insulin is a hormone that allows glucose to enter your cells so that you can obtain energy from the sugar. Type 1 diabetes is a chronic autoimmune condition in which the pancreas produces too little insulin or stops producing insulin completely. Without insulin glucose cannot enter the cells, so the sugar remains in the bloodstream, accumulating to abnormal levels, and the cells start to starve. A person with type 1 diabetes needs to take insulin, usually through injections or orally to allow glucose to enter into the cells.

Identifying Ketoacidosis

The signs of ketoacidosis generally appear within 24 hours of the accumulation of toxic ketone levels. Symptoms may include excessive thirst, increased urination, nausea, vomiting, abdominal pain, shortness of breath, weakness, fatigue, and confusion. The presence of ketones will make the breath smell fruity or ammonia-like (although this alone isn't a sign of ketoacidosis—those in nutritional ketosis may also experience fruity-smelling breath). Ketoacidosis is also characterized by a high level of ketones in the urine and high blood sugar.

Ketoacidosis is a medical emergency. If left untreated it can lead to loss of consciousness, coma, and even death. If you experience any of the signs and symptoms of ketoacidosis, seek medical attention immediately.

Insulin Resistance and Diabetes

A major component to keeping yourself healthy or improving any current health problems is regulating your blood sugar and insulin levels. Imbalances in blood sugar and insulin are significant factors in the rapidly growing epidemic in diabetes in both children and adults.

You already know that insulin is responsible for bringing the glucose from your bloodstream into your cells so that your body can use it as energy, but insulin also stimulates your liver and muscles to store excess glucose, which is called glycogen, for later use. In a healthy person insulin and glucose do their jobs effectively and efficiently, and as a result both insulin and glucose levels remain within a certain healthy range.

Insulin resistance is a condition in which the pancreas produces enough insulin, but the body does not use it effectively. When you're repeatedly exposed to high levels of insulin, your cells begin to say no thank you and start building up a resistance to insulin. When insulin, which carries glucose on its back, can't enter the cells, glucose remains in the bloodstream as well. This signals the pancreas to release even more insulin, which only exacerbates the cycle. While your body may be able to sustain this added stress for a certain period of time, eventually the pancreas gives up, and insulin production decreases or stops altogether.

Without insulin glucose can't enter the cells, so it stays in the bloodstream, wreaking havoc on your system. This is the point when many people are diagnosed with prediabetes or type 2 diabetes. Elevated glucose levels also contribute to obesity, high blood pressure, heart disease, certain types of cancer, and neurodegenerative disorders such as Alzheimer's disease.

Stay Alert

Many people aren't aware that they have insulin resistance until they are officially diagnosed with prediabetes or type 2 diabetes. Early warning signs of insulin resistance include fatigue, energy crashes, carbohydrate cravings, and weight gain around the midsection. If you experience any of these warning signs, it may be beneficial to have your insulin and glucose levels tested.

What's Carbs Got to Do with It?

When you eat carbohydrates, your body breaks them down into glucose. The rate at which this happens differs depending on the type of carbohydrates you're eating, but eventually all carbohydrates, with the exception of fiber, become glucose. When glucose enters your bloodstream, it triggers the release of insulin, as you already know. Constantly bombarding your body with carbohydrates and refined sugars increases glucose and insulin levels dramatically, increasing your risk of developing insulin resistance and the other resulting health problems. The goal is to avoid surges and crashes in glucose and insulin and to keep your levels consistent and steady throughout the day. When you do this, your body is better able to handle both glucose and insulin over the long term.

How Fat Can Help

Unlike with carbohydrates and refined sugars, eating fat doesn't cause a dramatic spike in glucose or insulin levels. When you turn your body from burning glucose for fuel to burning fat for fuel, which is the basis of the ketogenic diet, you help stabilize your glucose and insulin levels, which decreases your chances of developing insulin resistance.

Lack of Nutrients

In addition to the confusion between ketosis and ketoacidosis, opponents of the ketogenic diet have several other concerns about its safety. Many of these concerns arise from confusion about what the ketogenic diet actually is. Others are common myths that have been circulating for decades, yet are not backed by scientific literature.

One of the biggest concerns about the ketogenic diet is whether you'll be getting enough nutrients to keep you healthy. Opponents argue that you need a large amount of carbohydrates in your diet to stay healthy and that removing them prevents you from getting all the nutrients you need, but the benefits of carbohydrates, especially grains, are actually overstated.

It is true that your brain needs glucose to function, but your liver can make all of the glucose your brain needs from glycogen stored in the liver. If necessary your body can also obtain glucose from the protein you eat. A properly planned ketogenic diet supplies all of the nutrients your body needs to stay healthy and to run efficiently. A particular nutrient of concern is vitamin C since the richest sources of vitamin C are not permitted on a ketogenic diet; however, a properly planned ketogenic diet, which includes high-quality meat and lots of green vegetables, supplies all of the vitamin C you need.

Heart Disease

On the other end of the spectrum opponents of the ketogenic diet are also concerned that the diet is just too high in certain nutrients—fat and cholesterol, specifically. The belief is that eating too much fat will eventually lead to high cholesterol in the blood and result in heart troubles such as heart attack and heart disease. As previously mentioned, however, there is a great deal of confusion regarding what causes heart disease and whether fat plays as big a role as many believe it does. The quick answer to this is that scientific evidence does not support the theory that increased dietary fat intake leads to high blood cholesterol levels and heart disease.

This may come as a big surprise, especially if you've been told the opposite all your life, but to understand this concept you need to understand cholesterol. Cholesterol is not a bad thing. In fact it's necessary for survival. Cholesterol acts as a precursor to important hormones, including estrogen and testosterone. Your body uses cholesterol to make vitamin D, which plays a role in immune and neuromuscular function, moderates cell growth, and helps maintain calcium levels. Cholesterol also makes up the outer coating of each one of your cells. Without cholesterol you couldn't live.

On average the human body contains about 1,000 milligrams of cholesterol at any given time. Most of this cholesterol, about 75 percent, is actually made in the body by your liver. The rest, or 25 percent, comes from the food you eat. Because your body likes to keep cholesterol within a certain range and does a really good job of regulating it, the amount of cholesterol your liver produces varies based on how much cholesterol you eat. When you eat a lot of dietary cholesterol, the amount of cholesterol your body makes decreases. When the amount of cholesterol in your diet drops, your liver amps up production.

So, what about saturated fat? Although it's likely you've heard that saturated fat increases cholesterol levels and thus your risk of heart disease, most long-term studies have shown that this is not the case. In fact one study published in the journal *Obesity Reviews* in 2012 reported that a diet that is high in saturated fat (and low in carbohydrates) actually lowers the risk of developing heart disease by decreasing triglyceride levels, improving blood pressure, decreasing body mass index, and increasing HDL, or good cholesterol.

Kidney Problems

Because the ketogenic diet is low in carbohydrates, many assume that it's a high-protein diet (as previously mentioned it's actually a high-fat, moderate-protein diet), and there's a common misconception that eating too much protein can damage the kidneys. While it's true that those with damaged kidneys cannot handle protein as well as those with healthy kidneys, a high-protein diet will not damage the kidneys in otherwise healthy individuals.

There is the potential for kidney stones when following a ketogenic diet. In most cases kidney stones develop as a result of dehydration. To reduce the risk of developing kidney stones always make sure you're drinking enough water—at least half your body weight in ounces. If you have kidney trouble talk with your doctor before starting a ketogenic diet, as it may not be right for you.

When the Ketogenic Diet Should Not Be Used

While the ketogenic diet is safe for most individuals, there are some people who should not follow the diet plan. If you have certain metabolic conditions or health conditions, talk to your doctor before starting a ketogenic diet.

Contraindicated health conditions include:

- Gallbladder disease
- Impaired fat digestion
- History of pancreatitis
- Kidney disease
- Impaired liver function
- Poor nutritional status
- Previous gastric bypass surgery
- Type 1 diabetes
- Impaired insulin production
- Excessive alcohol use
- Carnitine deficiency
- Porphyria

On the other hand there are other groups of people for whom the ketogenic diet doesn't pose any serious health risks, but it may not necessarily benefit them either.

For people with metabolic disorders ketogenic diets pose more risk than benefit and can cause a great deal of harm. If you have one of these conditions, or if you drink alcohol excessively, a ketogenic diet is not for you.

Pregnancy and the Keto Diet

If you're pregnant or trying to become pregnant, a ketogenic diet may not be right for you. A woman is the most fertile when her body feels satisfied and well nourished. Because ketosis is essentially a starvation state, it's a gamble for women trying to become pregnant to try this diet. A high level of ketones in the blood may also pose a risk to a developing fetus. While traditional low-carbohydrate diets are okay during pregnancy, you should not limit your carbohydrates to the point of ketosis if you're pregnant.

High-Intensity Metabolic Conditioning

There are some conflicting views on whether following a ketogenic diet during periods of intense exercise is beneficial or not. Some athletes claim that ketosis boosts energy, while others, usually those who do high-intensity exercises such as sprints or CrossFit workouts, become burned out faster.

High-intensity exercises require glucose, and although your body can make glucose from protein and fat, it doesn't do it at the rate at which you need it to sustain high-intensity workouts. Because of this your body may turn to stored muscle glycogen, which depletes fairly quickly, and your performance may decrease. When you're burned out and your glycogen stores are depleted, you're more likely to have compromised form and sustain an injury during a workout.

Testing Your Ketone Levels

Once you've entered a state of ketosis, the goal is to stay there. The longer you remain in ketosis, the better your body gets at burning ketones for fuel and the better you'll feel. Testing your ketones will also allow you to monitor your ketone levels so that you'll know if they're getting too high. You can determine whether you're in ketosis and monitor your ketone levels using several different at-home test options.

Urine Test

Most drugstores carry urine strips that measure the amount of ketones in your urine. These urine strips test the pH of your urine and can give you a general idea of the level of ketones; however, they have their limitations.

There are three major types of ketones present in the blood when you've reached a state of ketosis: acetoacetate (AcAc), BHB, and acetone, which is a by-product of AcAc. After a few weeks on the ketogenic diet, levels of ketones begin to rise, and your body starts to use them as fuel. Once you become keto-adapted, which takes another few weeks, the muscles convert AcAc ketones into BHB ketones. So, why does this matter? The urine ketone test strips only measure for AcAc ketones, so while they're great for measuring your ketone levels when you're new to a ketogenic diet, they might not give you an accurate picture as your body becomes adapted to using ketones as fuel.

Also, as you become keto-adapted and your body begins to efficiently use ketones as fuel, you'll excrete fewer ketones in your urine. This means that a urine ketone test may show no ketones at all, even though you're actually in the optimal state of ketosis. Changes in hydration status also affect the amount of ketones in your urine. A high water intake will lower the concentration of ketones in the urine. Because it's important to stay well hydrated on a ketogenic diet, you may see numbers that don't give you an accurate picture.

Blood Test

Because urine testing is not as accurate over the long term, many people who are serious about staying in ketosis have turned to blood meters to test ketones. To test your blood ketone levels you'll prick your finger with a lancet, which is included in the blood meter kit, and then place a drop of blood on a specialized testing strip. The testing strip goes into the blood meter and gives you a reading on the screen.

Interpreting the Numbers

It's best to measure your blood ketone levels in the morning on an empty stomach since certain things—for instance, a high-fat meal—can affect the reading. A blood ketone level of below 0.5 millimoles per liter (mmol/L) is not considered ketosis. Once you reach a blood ketone level of 0.5 mmol/L to 1.5 mmol/L, you've entered a state of light nutritional ketosis. Here it's likely that you'll experience some weight loss, but the effects won't be optimal. Optimal ketosis is defined as having a blood ketone level of 1.5 mmol/L to 3.0 mmol/L. This is the state recommended for maximum fat burning. Ketone levels higher than 3.0 mmol/L are not necessary, and this is where ketosis has the potential to become dangerous. There is also anecdotal evidence that having a ketone level higher than the optimal range may actually inhibit fat loss.

When to Test

When you test your ketone levels is at least as important as the method you use to test. Because ketone levels fluctuate throughout the day and after meals, you have to be strategic about when you test to get an accurate reading. High-fat meals, especially those that contain a lot of medium-chain triglycerides (MCTs), will have a direct effect on ketone levels, so avoid testing immediately after meals. Intense aerobic exercise will also increase ketone levels. As a general rule ketone levels tend to be lower in the morning than in the evening because of all the fat you eat during the day. Testing in the morning right when you wake up may give you the most accurate results.

For the most accurate long-term results it's a good idea to test your ketone levels around the same time every day. If you have trouble remembering, set an alarm on your phone or another mobile device or write yourself a note by your bedside to test your levels right when you wake up.

Make Sure You Eat Enough

A ketogenic diet is not about excessively restricting calories. Although you do have to stay within a certain caloric range depending on your individual characteristics, you always want to make sure you're eating enough. Restricting carbohydrates and calories too much can leave you feeling tired and moody and can hinder your weight-loss progress.

A ketogenic diet isn't about starving yourself; it's about providing yourself with all of the calories and nutrients you need while restricting carbohydrate intake. As you lose weight, you may have to adjust the amount of calories you need, so make sure to monitor your progress and reevaluate your diet plan whenever necessary.

Vary Your Food Choices

As with any other diet plan varying your food choices as much as possible will help ensure that you're getting all of the nutrients you need to stay healthy. If you eat the same thing over and over, day after day, you may not be getting a certain vitamin or mineral that you need. A ketogenic diet is more restrictive than other diet plans, but that doesn't mean you don't have options. Familiarize yourself with your options and vary your plate as much as possible.

Consider Supplements

Many people can get all of the nutrients they need through a balanced ketogenic diet. However, some individuals may need supplementation with specific nutrients. This largely depends on individual characteristics. If you feel that you're doing everything right, but you still don't feel great on a ketogenic diet, contact a functional medicine practitioner or a functional nutritionist. These healthcare practitioners will be able to do the appropriate testing to determine if you have any nutritional deficiencies or to identify any areas where your diet may be lacking. Based on this information a functional medicine practitioner will be able to recommend specific supplements for you.

There are certain supplements that tend to be the most popular for people who follow a ketogenic diet. Leucine and lysine are two amino acids that help support ketosis and allow you a little more wiggle room with your protein intake. Although vitamin D levels tend to be low in the American population as a whole, those who follow a ketogenic diet may be at a higher risk of becoming deficient. Taking coconut oil as a supplement, 1 to 2 tablespoons per day, can help you reach your fat goals and help prevent constipation while on the diet.

Troubleshooting Constipation

Constipation is a common concern for those on a ketogenic diet, especially those who are in the early stages. If you're experiencing constipation on a ketogenic diet, there are some steps you can take to get things moving again.

In addition to taking 1 to 2 tablespoons of coconut oil each day drink adequate amounts of water (half of your body weight in ounces). If you're 200 pounds, this means 100 ounces of water every day. You also need to make sure you're getting enough salt, which helps maintain water balance and replenish sodium levels. Constipation may also be a sign that your protein intake is too high and your fat intake isn't high enough.

Achieving success on a ketogenic diet may take some trial and error and a little bit of practice, but once you get into the routine and reach a state of optimal ketosis, your body will adjust accordingly. If you experience any uncomfortable symptoms or hit any roadblocks, contact a functional medicine doctor or a functional nutritionist who can help you troubleshoot and overcome any hurdles.

The Ketogenic Diet for Epilepsy

Seizures come in many forms. They may be characterized by violent shaking or simply staring off into space for an extended period of time. A seizure occurs when the nerve cell activity in the brain is disrupted for any particular reason. Those who experience recurrent seizures are often given a diagnosis of epilepsy. Epilepsy is not a disease but rather the name of a group of neurological disorders characterized by recurring seizures without a known cause.

Approximately 10 percent of people will have a seizure at some point in their lifetime. Of those 10 percent only 30 percent will have a second seizure. When the seizures occur frequently, and with no known underlying cause, it's called epilepsy.

The condition affects more than 65 million people in the world. Currently, there are many medications available to help treat epilepsy, but approximately 30 percent of people with epilepsy don't respond to these medications. Some epileptic individuals may even benefit from surgery, but one of the oldest and least invasive epileptic treatment therapies is the ketogenic diet. Researchers aren't entirely sure how a ketogenic diet helps epilepsy, but research shows that the diet may elicit biochemical changes that prevent and eliminate short circuits in the brain's signaling system that are responsible for the seizures.

The History of the Ketogenic Diet for Seizures

According to a report in the medical journal *Epilepsia* fasting-type diets have been used to treat seizures since as early as 500 B.C. The first modern use of starvation as a treatment for epilepsy occurred in 1911, when Dr. Guelpa and Dr. Marie, two physicians from Paris, treated twenty adults and children with epilepsy and found that their symptoms were less severe during periods of metabolic starvation. This research was crucial to the introduction of the ketogenic diet as a dietary therapy for epilepsy.

In 1921 Dr. Wilder, a physician from the Mayo Clinic, hypothesized that you could achieve the benefits of fasting through other means besides completely restricting food, which isn't sustainable for the long term. Dr. Wilder said that not only would the ketogenic diet be just as effective as fasting, but patients could follow the diet for a long period of time because it supplied most of the nutrients that the body needed.

A colleague of Dr. Wilder, Dr. Peterman, calculated the ratios of macronutrients and came up with a plan that allowed dieters 1 gram of protein per kilogram of body weight, 10–15 grams of net carbohydrates per day, and the remainder of their calories from fat. The diet was used as a major treatment therapy for epilepsy throughout the 1920s and 1930s with a high success rate. In a textbook published in 1972 Dr. Livingston from Johns Hopkins Hospital revealed the results of a ketogenic diet intervention that he tested on 1,000 children. He reported that 52 percent of participants had complete control of their seizures when following a ketogenic diet, while another 27 percent had a significant improvement in seizure control. At the time, physicians could find treatment plans and instructions on how to calculate meal plans in almost every textbook, but with a rise in availability of antiseizure medications the diet fell out of fashion. Medicine was thought to be the treatment of the future, so physicians and dietitians were no longer being trained in the diet, and fewer children were placed on it. Currently, the ketogenic diet is still available as a treatment option for children with epilepsy in some select hospitals, but it's not as widely accepted or as well understood by physicians as it was in the past.

Who It Is For

As with any medical therapy the ketogenic diet is not for everyone who experiences seizures. Doctors typically only recommend the ketogenic diet for children with difficult-to-control seizures (especially those with Lennox-Gastaut syndrome). At the medical centers that still use the ketogenic diet it's usually not implemented until at least two or three medications have been shown to be ineffective and usually is recommended only for those who would not benefit from surgery.

Medical ketogenic diets for epilepsy should only be done under close supervision of a trained physician or nutrition professional. The diet is usually begun in a medical setting over a period of three or four days so that the child can be monitored closely. During this time the physician monitors blood sugar levels and ketone levels and watches for any seizures.

Traditionally, the ketogenic diet has been used for children with difficult-to-treat myoclonic, atonic, and tonic-clonic seizures. Myoclonic seizures are brief, shock-like jerks in a muscle or a group of muscles. They typically don't last for more than a couple of seconds. Atonic seizures are characterized by a sudden loss of muscle strength. Someone having an atonic seizure may have a drooping eyelid or suddenly drop their head. A tonic-clonic seizure, which is also known as a grand mal seizure, is the type most people picture when they hear the word *seizure*. Tonic-clonic seizures are characterized by a stiffening of the muscles followed by loss of consciousness. After the loss of consciousness comes rapid, rhythmic jerking of the muscles, especially in the arms and legs. A tonic-clonic seizure typically lasts 1 to 3 minutes.

The Diet Breakdown for Epilepsy

A medical ketogenic diet is stricter than a nutritional ketogenic diet, with different macronutrient ratios. A typical medical ketogenic diet allows four times as much fat as protein and carbohydrate combined (called a 4:1 ratio), but some children are put on a 3:1 ratio, or a ketogenic diet that allows three times as much fat as protein and carbohydrate combined.

Because of its critical purpose a medical ketogenic diet meal plan must be calculated by a trained dietitian or nutritionist, and each food must be weighed out on a gram scale to make sure that the exact meal plan is being followed. Just one off-plan meal can throw a child out of ketosis and result in a seizure. A typical meal consists of a protein-rich food, a fruit or vegetable, and a source of fat, such as butter, heavy cream, or mayonnaise.

Assessing the Results

Because each person is unique, it's impossible to say with certainty whether or not the diet will help control seizures, but for those who do benefit there is usually an improvement in frequency and/or severity of seizures within the first ten weeks. Many children, especially those on more than one antiseizure medication, are able to reduce the amount of medication they take. Some children are able to discontinue the use of medication completely. If the diet is successful, it's typically used for a period of up to three years. If no improvement is seen within the first few months, the physician or nutritionist will usually recommend stopping the diet.

Several studies have shown that once children who have seen no improvement from multiple epileptic medications are put on a ketogenic diet, they experience significant results. Fifty percent of children on a ketogenic diet experience a 50 percent decrease in seizures; approximately 33 percent see an improvement of at least 90 percent; and 10 percent become seizure-free and are able to get off all medication.

Alzheimer's Disease and Ketosis

Your brain contains 100 billion nerve cells. Each nerve cell is interconnected with millions of other nerve cells. These nerve cells communicate with each other to perform hundreds of functions, including remembering, thinking, and learning new things. Alzheimer's disease occurs when part of these nerve networks in the brain gets destroyed. Researchers aren't exactly sure what causes the damage associated with Alzheimer's, but what they do know is that when the damage occurs the nerve cells can no longer do their jobs.

Alzheimer's disease is the most common type of dementia—a general term that describes a decline in mental ability that is severe enough to interfere with day-to-day life. Someone with Alzheimer's disease usually experiences difficulty learning new information, memory loss, behavior changes, mood changes, disorientation, difficulty speaking and swallowing, trouble walking, and suspicions about family and friends. Healthcare professionals tend to agree that a combination of physical exercise, mental/social activity, and a healthy diet improve the brain health in those with Alzheimer's, but there is some disagreement about what actually constitutes a healthy diet for the condition.

Alzheimer's disease is the sixth leading cause of death in the United States and the fifth leading cause of death in Americans over the age of 65. Between the years 1999 and 2014 the number of deaths due to Alzheimer's increased by 55 percent.

Some health organizations recommend a diet that's low in all fat, especially saturated fat, and high in carbohydrates from fruits, vegetables, legumes, and whole grains, which is the complete opposite of a ketogenic diet. So, what does the research say?

Recent studies have shown that Alzheimer's patients who follow a ketogenic diet may not only experience improvement in symptoms like cognition and memory but may also experience a slowing of mental and physical decline. There is still some question as to why, but researchers believe it's because Alzheimer's disease is characterized by an inability of the brain to transport glucose across the blood-brain barrier. As a result the cells in the brain become starved of sufficient glucose, which leads to neurodegeneration, or the dying of nerve cells in the brain. The solution then would be to supply the brain with a different form of energy: ketones.

A study published in 2009 in *Nutrition & Metabolism* reported that study participants with mild to moderate Alzheimer's disease who were given a ketogenic agent showed significant improvement in their symptoms. Another study published in 2010 reported that of 60 study participants with dementia who had medium-chain triglycerides (MCTs) added to their diets, 90 percent reported improvement in at least one group of symptoms, which included memory, thinking, social interaction, sleep, vision, and appetite.

Although there hasn't been enough specific research on ketogenic diets and Alzheimer's disease to make conclusive statements, the research to date is highly encouraging regarding the effect of MCTs and ketogenic agents on symptom improvement.

Can Ketosis Help Other Health Conditions?

Encouraged by the epilepsy and Alzheimer's study results researchers have also been studying the effects of the ketogenic diet and resulting ketosis on other health conditions. Currently, there's not enough evidence to determine whether ketogenic diets should be a widely recommended part of the treatment for other health conditions, but the results of these preliminary studies have also been extremely positive.

Keto Diet and Parkinson's Disease

Parkinson's disease belongs to a group of disorders called motor system disorders. In someone with Parkinson's the dopamine-producing cells in the brain become destroyed, and the production of the neurotransmitter dopamine declines. Dopamine controls muscular movement, permitting smooth and fluid motion. After 60 to 80 percent of the dopamine-producing cells in the brain are destroyed, the symptoms of Parkinson's, which include shaking, tremor, slowness of movement, stiffness, and trouble balancing, begin to appear.

In general Parkinson's disease begins between the ages of 50 and 65. Approximately 1 percent of people in that age population are affected by the motor system disorder.

A study published in the medical journal *Neurology* reported that Parkinson's patients may see an improvement in symptoms when following a ketogenic diet. In the study, which didn't include a control group, Parkinson's patients were instructed to follow a ketogenic diet. After 28 days on the diet all study participants reported moderate to very good improvements in symptoms.

Although it is not entirely clear how a ketogenic diet could help improve symptoms in people with Parkinson's disease, scientists theorize that the ketones may actually bypass the area in the brain that is damaged and provide much-needed energy to other areas in the brain. Another theory is that the ketones, which have an anti-inflammatory effect on the brain, may be able to mend damaged neurons.

Keto Diet and Cancer

In 1923 a German biochemist named Otto Warburg suggested that cancer is caused by disruptions in normal metabolic processes that result in cancer cells taking up large amounts of energy in the form of glucose and converting it to lactate to produce energy. At the time, the hypothesis was highly controversial, but more recently his theory, which is now deemed the Warburg effect, has gotten some attention.

Cancer cells feed on glucose, but unlike heart, muscle, and brain cells, which can adapt to obtaining energy from ketones, tumor cells can't get enough energy from ketones. As a result researchers hypothesized that following a ketogenic diet may starve cancer cells of the glucose they need to survive, and eventually they will die off. Like all good theories this one was put to the test on several different occasions.

The first finding of the possibility of a ketogenic diet to help cancer was reported in 1995. Researchers put two brain cancer patients on a ketogenic diet that consisted of 60 percent MCTs (the fats that are found in high concentrations in coconuts), 10 percent other fats, 20 percent protein, and 10 percent carbohydrates. Both patients had aggressive brain tumors that were not responsive to traditional treatments and had been given a poor prognosis. After they followed the diet for a period of time, brain scans showed that the tumors started to shrink.

Another study published in 2007 reported that sixteen brain cancer patients who were instructed to follow a ketogenic diet experienced improvement in symptoms and quality of life. A third study in 2010 reported that when a sixty-five-year-old brain cancer patient was put on a restricted ketogenic diet, she reported cancer remission and absence of symptoms.

Although there isn't enough evidence to make conclusive statements about the potential role of the ketogenic diet in brain cancer treatment, the studies are promising.

Keto Diet and Mitochondrial Disorders

Mitochondria are known as the energy powerhouses in your body. The mitochondria turn the nutrients from the food you eat into a compound called adenosine triphosphate, or ATP, which provides energy to all of your cells. In those with mitochondrial disorders the mitochondria are dysfunctional, and as a result the cells are denied the energy they need. Because the cells of the brain, muscles, heart, nervous system, and eyes demand the most energy, they are often the most significantly affected areas of the body in someone with a mitochondrial disorder. Possible symptoms may include muscle weakness, hearing impairment, intellectual disabilities, learning disabilities, visual impairment, respiratory disorders, and seizures. Because there is no cure for mitochondrial disorders, treatment focuses on alleviating symptoms and improving quality of life.

Proper nutrition is often the primary therapy for mitochondrial disorders, and because seizures are a common symptom, the ketogenic diet is often part of the treatment plan. There have been several studies that show that the ketogenic diet not only helps reduce seizures in those with mitochondrial disorders but also improves symptoms and overall quality of life.

Keto Diet and Amyotrophic Lateral Sclerosis (Lou Gehrig's Disease)

Amyotrophic lateral sclerosis, or ALS, became well known when baseball great Lou Gehrig was diagnosed with the extremely rare degenerative disease in 1939. After the diagnosis the condition became commonly known as Lou Gehrig's disease.

ALS is a progressive neurodegenerative disorder that attacks the nerve cells in the brain and the spinal cord. The disease specifically affects the motor neurons, which control voluntary muscle movement. As the motor neurons die, they are no longer able to send nerve signals to the muscle fibers. When that happens, it can cause muscle weakness, slurred speech, and difficulty swallowing and breathing. Eventually, the muscles begin to atrophy, or become smaller, and the person affected becomes weaker and weaker.

The exact cause of ALS is unknown, but researchers believe that disruptions in the mitochondria in the brain play a role and that changing the type and amount of energy produced in the mitochondria through changes in diet may help those with ALS.

Although there is no cure for the disease, preliminary animal studies have shown that mice that were fed a ketogenic diet experienced a greater reduction in symptoms than mice who weren't. Because these studies were done on mice and not humans, there is no way to say whether humans would benefit in the same way, but preliminary results are encouraging.

These conditions are serious, and the decision to begin a medical ketogenic diet should not be taken lightly. If you or your child is affected by one of these disorders, consider talking with your physician or a trained nutrition professional about starting a ketogenic diet. If you do decide to implement a medical ketogenic diet, make sure you're closely following the instructions of your healthcare professional to avoid any complications or nutritional deficiencies. You should never start a medical ketogenic diet on your own.

5

Ingredients for Healthy Keto Cooking

The following are some tips for cooking on the ketogenic diet. You'll find advice on how to choose the right foods for you, how to cook them and make delicious meals, and why some of these foods are ketogenic diet all-stars. Dig in!

Be Choosy with Bacon

Like commercially prepared sausage, bacon often contains added sugar in the form of maple syrup or brown sugar. Look for uncured varieties at the supermarket or ask your local butcher to track down some sugar-free bacon for you.

There are two different ways you can get your bacon. For the panfrying method: Place the bacon slices closely together in a cold frying pan. Cook over medium heat without moving the slices for about 5 minutes. The bacon should by then move easily and not be stuck to the bottom of the pan. Flip the bacon and cook for about 5 more minutes. Remove from the pan and drain on a paper towel. For the oven method: Preheat oven to 400°F. Place a rack on a baking sheet. Lay the bacon slices on the rack and bake for 10–15 minutes depending on desired doneness level.

Vegetable Staples

Zucchini is a good source of vitamin C and vitamin B_6, and at only 2.5 net grams of carbohydrates per cup it makes a great addition to any ketogenic meal. Because zucchini is extremely mild tasting, you can add it to any meal without significantly changing the flavor. Zucchini is a fantastic choice for high-fat, low-carbohydrate diets because it has a low carbohydrate content (low glycemic index) and it's full of potassium, a crucial mineral for heart health. Besides that, it also makes a fantastic substitute for pasta lovers looking for low-carbohydrate alternatives.

One cup of chopped broccoli contains only 6 grams of carbohydrates, half of which come from fiber. In addition to being low in carbohydrates broccoli is high in vitamin C, a nutrient that you definitely need when following a ketogenic diet.

Broccoli contains a high amount of sulforaphane, a compound that helps stimulate detoxification and may help reduce the risk for certain types of cancers. According to a report in the *Journal of Agricultural and Food Chemistry* raw broccoli provides more sulforaphane than cooked broccoli, because the cooking process binds the compounds, making it less accessible.

Learning about Erythritol

Erythritol is a naturally derived sugar substitute that looks and tastes like sugar but has almost no calories and a low glycemic load, which means it doesn't significantly affect your blood sugar levels. Erythritol comes in two forms, granulated and powdered, and can be used in place of sugar in any recipe, although it is only 70 percent as sweet.

A for Avocado

Avocados are the ketogenic dieter's dream. A single avocado contains almost 30 grams of fat and only 3 grams of net carbohydrates. You can easily increase the fat content of any meal by adding a few slices of avocado. Avocados are also high in fiber and potassium and can help lower your cholesterol and triglycerides levels.

While most people know that an avocado is full of healthy fats, they would be hard-pressed to tell you the avocado is actually a fruit. To be more specific the avocado is a berry.

The Wonder of Wasabi

Wasabi is a plant in the same family as horseradish, which is used in Japanese cuisine to accompany sushi dishes. The flavor is similar to horseradish, with a particular pungency that is mainly felt in your nose. Wasabi can be bought in powder and mixed with water to form a paste, or you can buy it directly in paste form ready to use. Keep it handy to add a little spice to any dish that is tasting a little bland.

The Coconut!

Coconuts are rich in a specific type of fat called medium-chain triglycerides (MCTs). Instead of circulating through the blood like other fats MCTs go straight to the liver, where they're burned for energy. Because your body doesn't store MCTs, eating them can help boost weight loss.

The coconut milk that comes in a box is full of preservatives and low in fat. Some sweetened varieties contain sugar or other sweeteners that increase carbohydrate content. Look for full-fat coconut milk in a can that contains only coconut milk or a combination of coconut milk and guar gum. Unfortunately, there is a bit of inconsistency when it comes to canned coconut milk. Some brands whip up nicely, while others seem to fall flat. If you've followed the directions closely and still can't get a nice whipped cream, try a different brand of coconut milk—and make sure it's full fat.

Coconut cream is the solid portion of the coconut milk you buy in a can. You can easily separate the cream from the milk by refrigerating a can of full-fat milk for a few hours. When it's chilled, open the can and scoop out the solid part on top—this is the coconut cream and the part that contains most of the fat. Save the milk that's left at the bottom for a smoothie or use it in another recipe.

Coconut oil is a staple in the ketogenic diet. The oil is resistant to high heat, so unlike olive oil it doesn't oxidize with high temperatures. Coconut oil also contains MCTs, a type of fat that can help boost metabolism.

Picking Pork Rinds

Pork rinds are a great snack when you are on the keto diet and can even be used as a crunchy coating for chicken. But all pork rinds are not created equal. When choosing pork rinds read the ingredient list and choose one that contains only pork skin and pork fat or pork skin and salt. You want to avoid pork rinds that are cooked in processed lard.

Check Your Spices

It may come as a surprise but many commercial spices contain sugar or hydrogenated fats. Don't assume that an ingredient, such as lemon pepper, is free of carbohydrates until you check the label. If it contains sugar, ditch it and find one that doesn't. When it comes to herbs and spices there are plenty of sugar-free options out there.

Instead of using a prepared taco seasoning mix, which often contains sugar, artificial ingredients, and preservatives, make your own. Simply combine about 1 tablespoon of chili powder with about 1 teaspoon of cumin and about ¼ teaspoon each of onion powder, garlic powder, oregano, salt, and pepper. You can adjust these proportions to your taste or add some red pepper flakes for a little kick.

The Versatile Portobello

Portobello mushrooms are larger, more mature versions of the common white mushroom. The portobello mushroom has a rich, meaty flavor and texture, and because of this it's often used as a substitute for meat in vegetarian recipes. Portobello mushrooms are low in carbohydrates and loaded with essential vitamins and minerals, such as thiamine, magnesium, vitamin B_6, and iron, making them the perfect vehicle for getting quality sources of fat and protein.

Outstanding Omega-3s in Salmon

A 4-ounce fillet of salmon contains just about 15 grams of fat. Most of this fat comes in the form of omega-3 fatty acids, which promote brain health and heart health and help protect against cancer and autoimmune diseases such as rheumatoid arthritis and lupus.

When buying smoked salmon please make sure you get either wild or sustainably farmed. Often, conventionally farmed salmon contains high levels of antibiotics. Antibiotics from industrially farmed animals contribute to the creation of antibiotic-resistant superbugs.

While lox is generally a salted, not smoked, salmon, it is a popular way to serve salmon with cream cheese. Lox became a popular staple with Jewish immigrants in the late 1800s in America, but the mystery of when it was first combined with cream cheese, capers, red onion, and a bagel still remains.

Soy-Free Coconut Aminos

Coconut aminos sauce is a soy-free seasoning alternative made from the sap of coconut blossoms that you can use in place of soy sauce in any of your recipes. There is absolutely no coconut flavor—it tastes just like soy sauce, but unlike soy sauce, which is highly processed and most likely contains genetically modified organisms (GMOs), coconut aminos is GMO-free and contains 17 amino acids, vitamins, and minerals. Coconut aminos is a great substitution for soy sauce for people who prefer not using any soy products. Coconut aminos can be purchased through many major retailers online and in stores.

Stocking Up on Chicken

Chicken thighs are regularly on sale because they are less popular than chicken breasts. Take advantage of these sales by buying several packages at a time and freezing them for later. You can even cook the chicken before freezing to save time when making recipes down the road.

You can easily make your own chicken broth by covering about 3 pounds of chicken bones with water in a slow cooker and letting it simmer on low for at least 12 hours. Many commercial chicken broths contain unhealthy ingredients and preservatives, and while homemade chicken broth doesn't last as long, it's better for you.

European Delights

Mascarpone is an Italian soft cheese best known for being used in the famous tiramisu. It is actually the perfect ingredient for fat bombs; it's creamy, delicious, and contains zero carbs.

Crème fraîche is the French version of sour cream. Just like sour cream it is a cultured cream, but it has lower acidity and higher fat content, which makes it the perfect ingredient for fat bombs.

Try using both of these ingredients in the kitchen when you are in need of a fat boost.

A Note on Herbs

Cilantro is highly noted for its ability to act as a natural cleansing agent. The chemical compounds in cilantro bind to toxic metals such as mercury and help remove them from the body. Cilantro also acts as a strong antioxidant and may reduce the risk of heart disease.

Parsley isn't just a garnish. The herb is rich in vitamin C and vitamin A, so it helps keep your immune system, bones, and nervous system strong. Parsley also helps flush out excess water from the body and keeps your kidneys healthy.

You can substitute dried herbs for their fresh counterparts, but keep in mind that dried herbs are more concentrated, so they have a stronger flavor. If you choose to use dried herbs instead of fresh, use only ⅓ of the fresh amount. For example if the recipe calls for 3 tablespoons of fresh herbs, use only 1 tablespoon of dried herbs.

The Fishy Truth

If you're concerned about the mercury in tuna, keep in mind that adults can safely eat 18–24 ounces of tuna per month without a significant amount of mercury getting into their systems. If you'd like, swap out the tuna for canned salmon. Canned salmon is higher in omega-3 fatty acids and contains no mercury.

Looking for other fish to eat on your keto diet? Shrimp is an unusually concentrated source of the carotenoid astaxanthin, which acts as an antioxidant and an anti-inflammatory agent. Shrimp is also an excellent source of the mineral selenium.

Another fish you may want to try is Riga sprats. They are a delicacy imported from Latvia. They are a kind of small, oily fish (*Sprattus sprattus*) from the same family as the sardine. Riga sprats are smoked and preserved in oil. They are tender and flavorful and make the perfect base for a fat bomb!

Go Green with Asparagus and Brussels Sprouts

Asparagus is loaded with chromium, a trace mineral that enhances the activity of insulin, helping the hormone deliver glucose more efficiently from the bloodstream into your cells.

Serving for serving, Brussels sprouts contain significantly more vitamin C than an orange. They're also rich in vitamin A, beta-carotene, folic acid, iron, magnesium, selenium, and fiber. Chinese medicine practitioners often recommend Brussels sprouts to help with digestive troubles.

Picking a Probiotic

There are so many probiotics available that it can be difficult to know which one to pick. Choose a probiotic that contains at least seven different strains of bacteria and at least five billion organisms per dose. Make sure to store the probiotic per the manufacturer's instructions, as exposure to high heat and too much light can kill the bacteria, rending the probiotic useless.

Show Olives Some Love

The monounsaturated fats found in olives have been shown to encourage weight loss by breaking down the fats inside your fat cells and reducing insulin sensitivity. At only 1 gram of carbohydrates for five olives, they are a perfect ketogenic diet treat.

Tapenade is a fancy French word for a basic olive spread usually consisting of olives, capers, and anchovies. Anchovies provide great flavor and healthy omega-3s. You can always skip them if you do not enjoy the flavor.

Eggplant Trivia

Did you know that there are male and female eggplants? The male eggplants have fewer seeds than the female eggplants, so they tend to be less bitter. You can determine the sex of an eggplant by looking at the indentation on the bottom. If the indentation is shallow and round, it's a male; if the indentation is deep and more rectangular, it's a female.

Eggplant is a great meal when you're on the keto diet. Try baking the eggplant with a little Parmesan cheese. Parmesan cheese is aged so long that the proteins in it start to break down before it hits your digestive system. Much of the protein in it has already been broken down into peptides and free amino acids before you eat it—making digestion easier on you.

The Great Granola Debate

While many health food lovers believe granola to be an excellent nutrient-packed snack, others in the nutrition industry believe otherwise. Traditional granola, though full of fiber and iron from the rolled oats as well as healthy fats from the seeds and nuts, is also filled with alarming amounts of sugar, making it a less than healthy choice. You will be better off just turning to a handful of nuts for a quick snack that will keep your hunger pangs under control.

Green Rocket Fuel

Matcha is a finely ground powder of a specially grown green tea. Matcha is basically a form of whole green tea leaves with extra theanine and chlorophyll. It also contains high levels of catechin antioxidants and a good amount of caffeine. As matcha contains the whole leaf, you also get fiber and a higher content of nutrients than in regular brewed green tea.

Some of the many benefits of this antioxidant-rich powdered tea originating from Japan include enhanced energy, better concentration, and more endurance.

Go Nuts

When buying nuts opt for raw, unsalted varieties rather than roasted, salted, or sugared versions. Raw nuts generally contain no added ingredients, while roasted, flavored nuts can contain unhealthy oils and sugar.

Macadamia nuts have grown so much in popularity that California decided to get in on the growing action in the late 1980s. While the trees take four to five years to produce the nuts, they were an excellent investment for the warm climate in the southwestern states. Hawaii, however, is still the largest producer of these tasty nuts.

Pecans are one of the most antioxidant-rich tree nuts. They also contain more than nineteen vitamins and minerals, including vitamin A, folic acid, magnesium, potassium, and zinc. To presoak the pecans just leave them out on the counter overnight in warm water, and they will be ready to use in the morning.

One-half cup of pistachios provides 5 percent of your copper needs for the entire day. Copper is an essential trace mineral that plays an important role in metabolism and the formation of red blood cells.

Cashews have a lower fat content than most nuts, but that does not mean they're not a great addition to the ketogenic diet. Cashews are high in heart-healthy monounsaturated fats, such as those found in olive oil, and have been found to reduce high triglycerides in the blood. In general nuts promote heart health and lower the risk of weight gain, so add more servings to your diet to live your best!

No Ice Cream Maker? No Worries!

Making your own keto-friendly ice cream is a staple of the keto diet. Store-bought ice cream is loaded with sugar and artificial ingredients. Even if you don't have an ice cream maker, you can still enjoy homemade ice cream. Pour the mixed ingredients into a stainless steel bowl and put in the freezer for about 20 minutes. Once the edges of the mixture start to freeze, whisk the mixture rapidly until smooth and creamy. Repeat this every 20–30 minutes until ice cream forms.

A Little about Prosciutto

Prosciutto is made from the hind leg of a pig, or the ham. It is sliced thinly and rubbed with salt, which draws out the moisture to concentrate the flavor. This process, called curing, can take a few months to several years. To make easy prosciutto crumbles simply bake them in the oven. Preheat oven to 350°F. Place the thin prosciutto slices on a cookie sheet and bake them for about 12 minutes. Remove from the oven and let cool. Once cold and crispy, chop finely with a sharp kitchen knife until reduced to crumbles.

Chicken Skin Crisps

You can either buy chicken thighs and remove the skin to make your chicken skin crisps, or you can ask your local butcher or farmer from the farmers' market to sell you just chicken skin. You will be surprised; chicken skin is not so hard to find, and it will make superb crisps to use instead of crackers.

When you cook the chicken skins, you will end up with a pan full of chicken fat. You can drain that into a glass jar and save it for later. This fat can be stored in the refrigerator for a couple of months, and it can be used in any recipe as a 100 percent dairy-free substitute for butter.

Make Your Own

Coconut butter isn't always easy to find. It's simple and more cost-effective to make your own. To make 2 cups of coconut butter put 6 cups of unsweetened coconut flakes into a blender with a pinch of salt and blend until completely smooth. This usually takes 5–6 minutes. Making your own almond butter is simple and a great way to ensure that it doesn't contain any hidden sugar. Simply put almonds in a food processor and process until the oils break down and a nut butter forms. To up the fat content and make the almond butter smoother, add a couple of teaspoons of almond oil (or another oil of your choice).

Making cashew butter is the same basic process. To make about 1½ cups of cashew butter put 2 cups of unroasted, unsalted cashews in a food processor with a pinch of salt and 1 tablespoon of coconut oil. Process for about 30 seconds and then scrape down the sides of the food processor. Continue processing until smooth, scraping the sides when necessary. Be patient as the process can take several minutes.

Be Careful with Berries

Berries are full of fiber, so their net carbohydrate count is not as high as some other fruits. In fact, 1 cup contains 7 net carbohydrates. You still need to be careful when eating berries on a ketogenic diet. Don't overdo it and always make sure to count your macronutrients to make sure that berries fit into your plan that day.

Freeze-dried raspberries are a genius invention for cooking. They are relatively low in carbohydrates for a fruit and give a big punch of flavor.

Use What You've Got

When it comes to easy cooking the best way to reduce how much time you spend in the kitchen is to be prepared and to have the right tools. For example silicone molds are extremely helpful when you're on a ketogenic diet, especially if you're planning to make fat bombs a regular part of your diet. If you don't want to purchase silicone molds, you can use ice cube trays, but it will be harder to remove the bombs from the tray.

Turn Up the Heat

The capsaicin in chili peppers is thermogenic, which means it generates heat by increasing the metabolism of adipose, or fat, tissue. Eating capsaicin-rich foods may help stimulate the body's ability to burn fat.

Jalapeño peppers can vary greatly in their degree of heat. In the same batch you can find quite mild ones and some very spicy ones. Even if you like it hot, start your recipes without the seeds. You can always add heat, but you can't remove it!

Cayenne has the ability to promote a digestive enzyme that works to kill bad bacteria ingested from foods while promoting the good bacteria that optimizes the digestive process. You would think that such a spicy addition would cause stomach discomfort, but this pepper has amazing benefits. Cayenne also fights off the bad bacteria that cause stomach ulcers!

Turmeric and Cinnamon: Healing Spices

The main active ingredient in turmeric, called curcumin (not to be confused with the common spice cumin), is recognized as being a powerful anti-inflammatory. Even a small serving in a dish can assist your body's ability to digest fats and reduce bloating. It's also used medicinally to provide relief to sufferers of joint pain and swelling.

Filled with antioxidants, and anti-inflammatory in nature, cinnamon makes an excellent addition to any diet. Cinnamon is known to curb hunger, lower blood pressure, and reduce the risk of heart disease.

Soup Talk

If your soup is too salty, put a piece of raw potato in the soup or add a spoonful each of cider vinegar and erythritol. If soup is too greasy, drop in a lettuce leaf then take it back out after 2 minutes. The leaf will take some grease along with it. To create a thicker soup remove some of the cooked vegetables from the broth and purée them in a blender then stir them back into the soup. Or add full-fat coconut milk for an even richer soup.

Slow Cooker Tips

Use a rough sponge to remove any dried-on food from the slow cooker when cleaning it. A scouring pad could scratch the surface, creating a place for bacteria to grow. Store the slow cooker with the lid alongside instead of on top, to prevent the chance that mold will grow if you don't use it for several weeks.

Whey, Chia, and Flaxseed: What to Watch For

Although protein is the major nutrient in protein powders, a lot of them contain sweeteners that add a significant amount of carbohydrates. When choosing a protein powder look for one that is low in net carbohydrates and doesn't contain artificial ingredients.

Organic, nonorganic, ground, and whole flaxseed can be found in grocery aisles with nuts or near produce. You can purchase the whole seed product and use them in sandwiches, salads, and main dishes by using a coffee grinder to grind them until thoroughly powdered.

Additionally, a single ounce of chia seeds contains 9 grams of fat (5 of which are omega-3s) and 4 grams of protein. There are 12 grams of carbohydrates in an ounce, but since 11 of them come from fiber, an ounce of chia seeds clocks in at only 1 net carb, making them a ketogenic diet superfood.

Honeydew and Cantaloupe: Sweet Treats

Honeydew melon is related to the cantaloupe, but it has a smooth green flesh and a slightly milder flavor. Both fruits are often served for dessert. You can consume more than half of the recommended daily amount of vitamin C with just one wedge of honeydew melon; one wedge of cantaloupe will provide over 100 percent of the recommended daily amount of vitamin C and 120 percent of vitamin A.

Fiber Benefits

Leafy greens, vegetables, and fruits all contain some amount of this miracle substance. Because the human body is almost completely unable to digest fiber, we benefit from its tendency to make our stomachs feel full and to clear our intestinal tracts by remaining nearly intact throughout digestion. Although fiber is available in pill and powder forms, those are a far cry from a healthy bowl of spinach or broccoli.

Oranges and Limes: The Power of Vitamin C

Oranges are well known for their immunity-building power, and rightfully so! Consuming oranges every day can help the human body fight off illnesses from the common cold to serious cancers and heart disease. You can thank the rich beta-carotene and the vitamin C. An orange is a definite must for health and longevity.

Although many patients suffering from arthritis decide to exercise and eat differently, few know the powerful effects limes can have on joints! These vitamin C–filled fruits can pack a punch in reducing arthritis symptoms to a minimum and making everyday life seem less achy!

Hemp Hearts

Hemp hearts are the shelled seeds of the hemp plant. They do not contain any psychoactive compounds, but they do contain a lot of great omega-3s. They are becoming more and more popular because of their great nutrient content and sustainable origin. They have great macros for a fat bomb: per 30-gram serving, hemp hearts contain 10 grams of plant-based protein and 10 grams of omega-3s.

Healing Power of Ginger

Ginger is not only a delicious flavor for both sweet and savory dishes, but it is also a medicinal root. It has great digestive properties, it prevents gas, and it is most effective at eliminating nausea. If you are feeling a little nauseated, try adding two or three slices of gingerroot to hot water with a squeeze of lemon. Let the mixture steep for a few minutes until the flavors have melded. Sip until you are feeling better!

Make It a Paste

Ginger garlic paste is a great flavor addition for savory meals and fat bombs. To make this versatile paste combine 4 ounces of chopped garlic and 4 ounces of fresh peeled and chopped gingerroot in a food processor. While pulsing, slowly drizzle in one tablespoon of olive oil. Continue pulsing until a smooth paste forms. Store the paste in an airtight jar in the refrigerator. The paste will keep for up to 2 weeks in the refrigerator.

Food Flavoring versus Sugar-Free Syrup

A lot of recipes on the ketogenic diet call for sugar-free syrup. Such syrups contain ingredients like acesulfame potassium, sodium hexametaphosphate, or phosphoric acid. Those artificial flavors, preservatives, and fillers are not health-building ingredients; on the contrary they load the body with toxins, which make it much harder to lose unwanted pounds. A good organic maple flavor will only contain a maple distillate and pure grain alcohol in minimal quantities.

6

50+ Ketogenic Recipes

Here are more than fifty ketogenic recipes that are flavorful, easy to make, and delicious!

Bacon-Wrapped Egg Cups

To give this recipe a little kick, replace the Cheddar cheese with pepper jack and add a pinch of red pepper flakes to the eggs while you're whisking.

Serves 12

12 slices sugar-free bacon
12 large eggs
½ cup heavy cream
½ teaspoon salt

¼ teaspoon freshly ground black pepper
½ cup shredded Cheddar cheese
2 cups chopped and steamed broccoli

1. Preheat oven to 350°F.
2. Cook bacon in a medium skillet over medium heat until almost crisp. When bacon is fully cooked, quickly line each well of a greased 12-cup muffin tin with a piece of bacon.
3. Whisk eggs, heavy cream, salt, and pepper together in a large mixing bowl. Add cheese and chopped broccoli and stir.
4. Pour an equal amount of mixture into each well of the muffin tin.
5. Bake for 20 minutes or until lightly browned on top and firm throughout.
6. Allow to cool for 10 minutes and then remove egg cups from muffin tins. Store in refrigerator.

PER SERVING	Fat: 13.1g	Sodium: 398mg	Carbohydrates: 2.6g
Calories: 187	Protein: 12.5g	Fiber: 0.9g	Sugar: 0.9g

Almond Butter Muffins

For some variation replace the almond butter in this recipe with another one of your favorite nut butters. Cashew butter, peanut butter, and sunflower seed butter work well.

Serves 12

⅔ cup almond flour
¼ cup granulated erythritol or granular
   Swerve
1 teaspoon ground cinnamon
¼ cup unsweetened almond butter

2 tablespoons unsalted butter
1 tablespoon coconut oil
1 teaspoon vanilla extract
4 large eggs
¼ cup heavy cream

1. Preheat oven to 350°F.
2. Mix together almond flour, granulated erythritol or Swerve, and cinnamon in a medium mixing bowl.
3. In a separate medium mixing bowl beat almond butter, butter, coconut oil, vanilla extract, eggs, and heavy cream together until smooth.
4. Add almond flour mixture to almond butter mixture and stir until smooth.
5. Put a paper cupcake liner in each well of a 12-cup muffin tin. Fill each paper cup with batter.
6. Bake for 20 minutes or until a toothpick inserted in the center comes out clean.
7. Remove from muffin tin and allow to cool before serving.

PER SERVING		
Calories: 112	Protein: 3.4g	Carbohydrates: 7.0g
Fat: 9.4g	Sodium: 42mg	Sugar: 0.4g
	Fiber: 1.5g	Sugar alcohol: 4.0g

Smoked Salmon and Brie Baked Avocado

Smoked salmon and Brie are a classic combination. These avocados are great served cold, but are so much better when hot and melted!

Makes 2 fat bombs

1 medium avocado, halved and pitted, skin on

1½ ounces wild-caught smoked salmon, coarsely chopped

1 tablespoon plus 1 teaspoon Brie cheese

¼ teaspoon freshly ground black pepper

1. Preheat oven to 350°F.
2. Place avocado halves hole-side up in a shallow ramekin or ovenproof dish just large enough to hold them.
3. Mix salmon, Brie, and pepper in a small bowl, then scoop ½ mixture into each avocado cavity.
4. Bake 20 minutes. Serve hot.

PER 1 FAT BOMB
Calories: 158

Fat: 11.7g
Protein: 6.5g

Sodium: 184mg
Fiber: 4.7g

Carbohydrates: 6.1g
Sugar: 0.2g

Savory-Sweet Baked Avocado with Pecans and Coconut

This is a recipe that mixes savory and sweet. It has a subtle sweetness but no added sugar.

Makes 2 fat bombs

1 medium avocado, halved and pitted, skin on

2 tablespoons grated unsweetened coconut

2 tablespoons coconut oil

6 pecan halves

1. Preheat oven to 350°F.
2. Place avocado halves hole-side up in a shallow ramekin or ovenproof dish just large enough to hold them.
3. Mix grated coconut with coconut oil in a small bowl and scoop into each avocado cavity.
4. Place 3 pecans on top of each avocado half, gently nudging them in.
5. Bake 20 minutes. Serve hot or cold.

PER 1 FAT BOMB	Fat: 27.7g	Sodium: 6mg	Carbohydrates: 7.5g
Calories: 285	Protein: 2.0g	Fiber: 5.5g	Sugar: 0.6g

Smoked Salmon Mousse Bacon Cups

The salty crunch of bacon surrounding a luscious, creamy salmon mousse is the definition of decadence. Intensifying the flavor with fresh herbs only adds to the gourmet taste of this fantastic finger food.

Makes 6 fat bombs

12 slices regular-cut sugar-free bacon, 6 cut in half

6 ounces wild-caught smoked salmon

4 ounces cream cheese, softened

1 tablespoon heavy whipping cream

⅛ teaspoon freshly ground black pepper

1 teaspoon fresh dill, plus 6 sprigs for garnish

1. Preheat oven to 400°F.
2. In a standard-sized muffin tin, place half-strips bacon in an X shape in the bottom of 6 cups.
3. Line those same cups with 1 full slice bacon along the inside of the cup vertically.
4. Place a cookie sheet underneath muffin tin and bake cups 12–15 minutes until slightly browned and crisp.
5. While cups are baking, combine remaining ingredients except for the sprigs of dill in a food processor and pulse until smooth. Cover and set in refrigerator to chill.
6. After bacon cups have cooled, fill with mousse mixture and serve with a fresh sprig of dill on top.

PER 1 FAT BOMB	Fat: 15.3g	Sodium: 647mg	Carbohydrates: 1.5g
Calories: 214	Protein: 14.2g	Fiber: 0.1g	Sugar: 0.7g

Sausage Quiche

This quiche holds up well in the fridge, so it's a good choice when meal planning. You can prepare the quiche on Sunday, put each serving in a plastic container in the fridge, and eat it for breakfast all week.

Serves 12

12 large eggs
¼ cup heavy cream
½ teaspoon salt
¼ teaspoon freshly ground black pepper

12 ounces cooked crumbled sugar-free breakfast sausage
2 cups shredded Cheddar cheese

1. Preheat oven to 375°F.
2. Whisk eggs, heavy cream, salt, and pepper together in a large bowl.
3. Add breakfast sausage and Cheddar cheese.
4. Pour mixture into a greased 9" × 13" casserole dish.
5. Bake for 25 minutes. Cut into 12 squares and serve.

PER SERVING	Fat: 18.9g	Sodium: 633mg	Carbohydrates: 2.0g
Calories: 262	Protein: 16.3g	Fiber: 0.0g	Sugar: 0.6g

Taste Enhancer!

You will find that once you reduce the amount of sugar you consume, your taste buds will reset. You'll start enjoying much wider nuances of flavor!

Ham, Cheese, and Egg Casserole

Mozzarella and Cheddar cheese give this dish a mild cheesy flavor, but you can use any type of shredded cheese you want.

Serves 6

4 cups broccoli florets

12 large eggs

2 cups cooked diced sugar-free ham

½ cup shredded mozzarella cheese

½ cup shredded Cheddar cheese

¼ cup chopped scallions

1. Preheat oven to 375°F.
2. Fill a large pot with water and bring to a boil. Blanch broccoli by putting in boiling water for 2–3 minutes.
3. Put eggs, ham, mozzarella, Cheddar, and scallions in a large bowl and whisk until combined. Add broccoli.
4. Pour into a 9" × 13" baking dish and cook for 35 minutes or until eggs are cooked through.

PER SERVING	Fat: 15.8g	Sodium: 893mg	Carbohydrates: 3.8g
Calories: 296	Protein: 30.1g	Fiber: 0.1g	Sugar: 0.6g

Bacon Cheddar Soup

If you don't have an immersion blender, you can pour the soup into the pitcher of a regular blender instead. Just make sure that it's not too hot, or you may have an explosive mess on your hands.

Serves 4

4 slices thick-cut sugar-free bacon
1 small onion, chopped
2 cloves garlic, minced
3 cups cauliflower florets
½ teaspoon dry mustard

½ teaspoon freshly ground black pepper
3 cups sugar-free chicken broth
2 cups heavy cream
2 cups shredded Cheddar cheese
1 tablespoon grated Parmesan cheese

1. Cook bacon over medium-high heat in a medium skillet until crisp, about 10 minutes.
2. Remove bacon from pan, reserving bacon grease. Return pan to heat.
3. Place onions and garlic in bacon grease and sauté until translucent, 3–4 minutes. Chop cauliflower florets into small pieces and add to onions and garlic. Sauté until tender, 7–10 minutes. Add dry mustard and black pepper and stir.
4. Transfer onions, garlic, cauliflower, and bacon grease to a large stockpot. Add chicken broth and heavy cream.
5. Stir all ingredients together and bring to a boil over medium heat. Once mixture begins to boil, reduce heat to a simmer.
6. Insert an immersion blender into the soup and blend until creamy. Add Cheddar cheese and Parmesan cheese and stir until melted.
7. Dice bacon and stir into soup. Serve hot.

PER SERVING			
Calories: 744	Fat: 62.7g	Sodium: 1,342mg	Carbohydrates: 12.6g
	Protein: 23.5g	Fiber: 2.2g	Sugar: 7.0g

Pumpkin Cream Soup

Instead of using cinnamon, nutmeg, and ginger in this recipe, you can use just over a teaspoon of pumpkin pie spice.

Serves 6

2 tablespoons coconut oil
2 tablespoons unsalted butter
¼ cup diced onion
2 cloves garlic, minced
3 cups sugar-free chicken broth
1½ cups pumpkin purée

½ teaspoon ground cinnamon
½ teaspoon ground nutmeg
⅛ teaspoon ground ginger
¼ teaspoon salt
¼ teaspoon freshly ground black pepper
3 cups full-fat canned coconut milk

1. Heat coconut oil and butter in a stockpot over medium-high heat. When oil and butter are hot, add onions and garlic and sauté until translucent, 3–4 minutes.
2. Add chicken broth, pumpkin purée, cinnamon, nutmeg, ginger, salt, and pepper and stir until combined.
3. Submerge an immersion blender into soup and blend until smooth and creamy. Allow to simmer for 20 minutes.
4. Stir in coconut milk. Serve hot.

PER SERVING			
Calories: 317	Fat: 30.7g	Sodium: 575mg	Carbohydrates: 7.1g
	Protein: 3.8g	Fiber: 1.5g	Sugar: 1.8g

Creamy Broccoli Soup

The creamy, nutty flavor of the coconut milk in this recipe complements the broccoli nicely, but if you don't like the coconut flavor, you can use heavy cream instead.

Serves 6

2 tablespoons unsalted butter
2 stalks celery, diced
1 medium onion, diced
6 cups broccoli florets

½ teaspoon salt
½ teaspoon freshly ground black pepper
4 cups sugar-free chicken broth
2 cups full-fat canned coconut milk

1. Heat butter over medium-high heat in a large stockpot. Add celery and onions and sauté until translucent, 3–4 minutes.
2. Add broccoli florets, salt, pepper, and chicken broth and bring to a simmer. Allow to simmer until broccoli is fork tender, about 10 minutes.
3. Add coconut milk and blend with an immersion blender until soup is smooth and creamy. Serve hot.

PER SERVING	Fat: 18.9g	Sodium: 850mg	Carbohydrates: 8.8g
Calories: 221	Protein: 5.1g	Fiber: 0.6g	Sugar: 1.7g

Be Choosy with Dairy

Choose grass-fed butter, raw cheese, and organic heavy cream whenever possible.

Ham and Cheese Casserole

Allow the cream cheese to reach room temperature before starting this recipe. Softened cream cheese is much easier to work with than cream cheese fresh from the fridge.

Serves 6

6 cups cauliflower florets
½ cup cream cheese, softened
½ cup heavy cream
¼ cup coconut cream
2½ cups cooked cubed sugar-free ham

1 cup shredded Cheddar cheese
1½ tablespoons grated Parmesan cheese
¼ cup chopped scallions
½ teaspoon salt
¼ teaspoon freshly ground black pepper

1. Preheat oven to 350°F. Bring a large pot of water to a boil and add cauliflower. Boil until cauliflower is fork tender, about 5–10 minutes. Strain cauliflower and return to pot.
2. Put cream cheese, heavy cream, and coconut cream in a medium mixing bowl and beat with a handheld beater until smooth. Transfer cream cheese mixture to cauliflower pot and stir until cauliflower is coated. Add in ham, Cheddar cheese, Parmesan cheese, scallions, salt, and pepper and stir until combined.
3. Transfer mixture to a 9" × 9" baking dish and bake until cheese is melted and casserole is bubbly, about 30 minutes. Serve hot.

PER SERVING	Fat: 23.6g	Sodium: 1,223mg	Carbohydrates: 7.8g
Calories: 355	Protein: 23.2g	Fiber: 2.3g	Sugar: 3.7g

Deli Roll-Ups

Instead of purchasing prepared chive cream cheese, you can make your own by combining plain cream cheese with minced onions and dried chives.

Serves 2

8 ounces sugar-free deli ham, sliced
½ cup chive cream cheese

1 cup chopped baby spinach
1 red bell pepper, sliced

1. Lay out each slice of ham flat. Take 1 tablespoon of cream cheese and spread it on a slice of ham. Repeat for the remaining slices.
2. Put 2 tablespoons of chopped spinach on top of the cream cheese on each slice.
3. Divide bell pepper into 8 equal portions and put each portion on top of spinach.
4. Roll up the ham and secure with a toothpick. Eat immediately or refrigerate until ready to serve.

PER SERVING	Fat: 19.7g	Sodium: 1,723mg	Carbohydrates: 5.2g
Calories: 302	Protein: 24.1g	Fiber: 0.8g	Sugar: 3.2g

Check Your Labels!

Many hams contain cane sugar, brown sugar, maple syrup, or honey. When choosing a ham read your labels carefully and stay away from any that contain added sugars, which will up the carbohydrate content of this meal significantly.

Chicken Cordon Bleu Casserole

Traditional chicken cordon bleu contains ham, chicken, and Swiss cheese, but if you're not a fan of Swiss cheese, swap it out for a cheese with a milder flavor, such as provolone or mozzarella.

Serves 4

2 cups cooked chopped boneless, skinless chicken breast
1 cup cooked diced sugar-free ham
1 cup cubed Swiss cheese
½ cup heavy cream
½ cup sour cream
½ cup cream cheese
½ teaspoon granulated garlic
½ teaspoon granulated onion
¼ teaspoon salt
¼ teaspoon freshly ground black pepper
1 ounce crushed pork rinds

1. Preheat oven to 350°F.
2. Mix chicken and ham and spread out in the bottom of a 9" × 13" baking dish.
3. Sprinkle Swiss cheese on top of chicken and ham.
4. Put heavy cream, sour cream, and cream cheese in a medium saucepan and heat over medium heat until cream cheese is melted and mixture is smooth. Add garlic, onion, salt, and pepper. Pour mixture over chicken, ham, and Swiss cheese.
5. Sprinkle pork rinds across casserole. Bake for 30 minutes, or until slightly browned and cheese is bubbly.

PER SERVING			
Calories: 584	Fat: 38.9g	Sodium: 927mg	Carbohydrates: 5.2g
	Protein: 44.0g	Fiber: 0.1g	Sugar: 3.1g

Homemade Mayonnaise

You can use olive oil in this recipe in place of avocado oil. If you prefer a milder taste, opt for extra-light olive oil. If you like mayonnaise with a strong olive oil flavor, go for extra-virgin.

Serves 10

1 large egg, room temperature
Juice from ½ lemon, room temperature
½ teaspoon dry mustard

½ teaspoon salt
¼ teaspoon freshly ground black pepper
1 cup avocado oil

1. Combine egg and lemon juice in a narrow container and let sit for 30 minutes.
2. Add dry mustard, salt, pepper, and avocado oil. Insert an immersion blender into mixture until it hits the bottom of the container.
3. Turn the blender on and blend for 30 seconds. As the mixture starts to emulsify, pull the blender out of the mixture slightly to mix in the oil on the top.
4. Transfer to a tightly sealed container and store in the refrigerator.

PER SERVING	Fat: 21.3g	Sodium: 123mg	Carbohydrates: 0.3g
Calories: 201	Protein: 0.7g	Fiber: 0.0g	Sugar: 0.1g

Creating an Emulsion

Mayonnaise is made by creating an emulsion, or a mixture of oil and water (from the eggs). As you know, oil and water do not mix easily, so it's important to let the egg and lemon juice reach room temperature before preparing this recipe. If you don't, the emulsion may fail, and you'll be left with a runny mess.

Ranch Dressing

You can easily add this dressing to salads, Deli Roll-Ups, and chicken dishes for a quick boost in fat content.

Makes 1½ cups (Serves 12)

1 cup Homemade Mayonnaise (see recipe in this chapter)
½ cup sour cream
½ teaspoon white vinegar
¼ cup chopped fresh parsley
2 tablespoons chopped fresh dill

½ teaspoon dried chives
¼ teaspoon garlic powder
¼ teaspoon onion powder
⅛ teaspoon salt
⅛ teaspoon freshly ground black pepper

Put all ingredients in a medium mixing bowl and whisk until smooth. Cover and refrigerate for at least 30 minutes before serving.

PER SERVING
Calories: 154

Fat: 15.9g
Protein: 0.8g

Sodium: 112mg
Fiber: 0.1g

Carbohydrates: 1.0g
Sugar: 0.4g

Avocado Italian Dressing

You can make this more of a traditional Italian dressing by using light olive oil in place of avocado. Give it an Asian kick by using toasted sesame oil instead.

Makes 1½ cups (Serves 12)

1 cup avocado oil
¼ cup white wine vinegar
3 tablespoons water
1 teaspoon garlic salt
1 teaspoon onion powder

2 teaspoons dried oregano
½ teaspoon dried basil
1 teaspoon dried parsley
1 teaspoon salt
1 teaspoon freshly ground black pepper

1. Whisk all ingredients together in a medium mixing bowl until combined.
2. Serve immediately or store at room temperature and shake or mix well before serving.

PER SERVING			
Calories: 163	Fat: 17.4g	Sodium: 357mg	Carbohydrates: 0.4g
	Protein: 0.1g	Fiber: 0.2g	Sugar: 0.0g

BLT Salad

The combination of flavors in this bacon, lettuce, and tomato salad is so delicious that you won't even miss the bread.

Serves 4

1 pound sugar-free bacon
1 head romaine lettuce
2 large tomatoes, diced
2 large avocados, diced

½ cup Homemade Mayonnaise (see recipe in this chapter)
1 tablespoon white vinegar

1. Cook bacon over medium-high heat in a large skillet until crisp, about 10 minutes. Remove from heat, allow to cool, and then roughly chop and put in a medium mixing bowl.
2. Roughly chop romaine lettuce. Add lettuce, tomatoes, and avocado to bacon and toss until combined.
3. In a separate medium mixing bowl combine mayonnaise and white vinegar. Pour mayonnaise mixture over bacon mixture and toss to coat. Refrigerate until chilled, about 30 minutes. Serve chilled.

PER SERVING			
Calories: 621	Fat: 51.7g	Sodium: 1,389mg	Carbohydrates: 13.7g
	Protein: 21.3g	Fiber: 7.9g	Sugar: 3.8g

Let It Sit

You can eat this salad as soon as it's chilled, or you can let it sit for a few hours or overnight to let the flavors develop. If you choose to let it sit overnight, leave the lettuce out and add it when you're ready to eat so that it stays crunchy.

Spinach and Prosciutto Salad

The unsalted cashews in this recipe help satisfy that craving for something crunchy when you're eating a salad. As a bonus, they taste great with avocado.

Serves 4

8 cups baby spinach
12 ounces prosciutto
2 large avocados, diced
½ cup diced red onion

½ cup chopped raw unsalted cashews
½ cup Avocado Italian Dressing (see recipe in this chapter)

1. Put spinach in a large mixing bowl. Dice prosciutto and put on top of spinach. Put diced avocado, red onions, and chopped cashews on top of spinach.
2. Add dressing to salad and toss to coat. Serve immediately.

PER SERVING

Calories: 430

Fat: 50.0g
Protein: 29.0g

Sodium: 2,235mg
Fiber: 7.3g

Carbohydrates: 20.6g
Sugar: 2.7g

Chef Salad

Meat and cheese are the basis of a Chef Salad. Although this recipe calls for ham and turkey and Swiss and Cheddar, you can use any combination you'd like. Try adding roast beef and some pepper jack for a little kick.

Serves 4

8 cups chopped romaine lettuce
1 cup diced sugar-free ham
1 cup diced turkey
1 cup cubed Swiss cheese
1 cup cubed Cheddar cheese

4 large hard-boiled eggs, sliced
½ cup crumbled sugar-free bacon
½ cup Ranch Dressing (see recipe in this
  chapter)

Combine all ingredients in a large bowl and toss to combine. Serve immediately.

PER SERVING	Fat: 48.4g	Sodium: 1,334mg	Carbohydrates: 7.3g
Calories: 700	Protein: 48.5g	Fiber: 2.1g	Sugar: 2.6g

Cheeseburger Salad

When you eat this salad, you get all the flavors of a cheeseburger without the insulin- and glucose-spiking bun.

Serves 4

1 pound 85/15 ground beef
½ teaspoon salt
¼ teaspoon freshly ground black pepper
⅓ cup sugar-free ketchup
1 tablespoon yellow mustard
1 teaspoon spicy brown mustard
1 head romaine lettuce

1 medium red onion, chopped
2 medium tomatoes, diced
4 dill pickle spears, cubed
1 cup shredded Cheddar cheese
½ cup Homemade Mayonnaise (see recipe in this chapter)
1 tablespoon white or apple cider vinegar

1. Brown ground beef in medium skillet over medium heat. Once beef is browned, add salt, pepper, ketchup, yellow mustard, and spicy mustard. Stir until combined. Remove from heat and set aside.
2. Chop romaine lettuce and put into a large mixing bowl. Top with onions, tomatoes, pickles, shredded cheese, and beef.
3. In a separate small mixing bowl, combine mayonnaise with vinegar and stir until smooth. Drizzle over salad and toss to coat. Serve immediately.

PER SERVING

Calories: 525	Fat: 38.9g	Sodium: 1,253mg	Carbohydrates: 11.2g
	Protein: 23.4g	Fiber: 3.9g	Sugar: 4.4g

Deviled Eggs

Deviled Eggs are a staple at any party, and they make the perfect ketogenic diet snack. Whip some up and store them in your refrigerator for when you need some fat and protein in a hurry.

Serves 6

6 large hard-boiled eggs
¼ cup Homemade Mayonnaise (see recipe
   in this chapter)
1 teaspoon white vinegar

1 teaspoon dry mustard
½ teaspoon salt
¼ teaspoon freshly ground black pepper
⅛ teaspoon smoked paprika

1. Peel eggs and cut in half lengthwise. Scoop out egg yolks and put in a small mixing bowl.
2. Mash yolks with a fork, then add mayonnaise, vinegar, mustard, salt, and pepper. Continue to mash until combined.
3. Divide mixture into 12 equal portions and fill each egg white half. Sprinkle with paprika.

PER SERVING
Calories: 146

Fat: 11.6g
Protein: 6.6g

Sodium: 296mg
Fiber: 0.1g

Carbohydrates: 0.9g
Sugar: 0.6g

Parmesan Chips

You can make this recipe with any type—or combination of types—of cheeses you want. Try Cheddar, pepper jack, or a combination of Parmesan and Cheddar.

Serves 4 (Makes 16 chips)

½ cup grated Parmesan cheese

½ cup shredded Parmesan cheese

1. Preheat oven to 375°F.
2. Mix grated and shredded Parmesan cheese together. Drop by the tablespoon onto parchment paper–lined baking sheets.
3. Bake for 5 minutes or until cheese is crisp and slightly browned.
4. Remove from oven and allow to cool. Peel chips off parchment paper and serve.

PER SERVING			
Calories: 94	Fat: 5.7g	Sodium: 395mg	Carbohydrates: 2.1g
	Protein: 7.3g	Fiber: 0.0g	Sugar: 0.1g

Jalapeño Poppers

To double the yield of this recipe, cut the jalapeños in half and wrap each half in a half piece of bacon.

Serves 4

8 jalapeño peppers
½ cup cream cheese, softened

½ cup shredded pepper jack cheese
8 slices sugar-free bacon

1. Preheat oven to 425°F.
2. Cut about ⅓ of each pepper off lengthwise to make a little pocket for filling. Scoop out seeds.
3. Mix cream cheese and pepper jack cheese together in a small bowl. Divide filling into 8 equal portions and stuff each pepper with cheese filling.
4. Wrap each pepper in bacon. Lay flat on a cookie sheet lined with aluminum foil and bake for 15–20 minutes, or until bacon is crispy.

PER SERVING	Fat: 20.6g	Sodium: 579mg	Carbohydrates: 3.8g
Calories: 270	Protein: 13.1g	Fiber: 0.8g	Sugar: 2.2g

Guacamole

Guacamole is a ketogenic diet staple. Eat it with some celery stalks, put it on top of your taco bowls, or spoon it right out of the bowl.

Serves 4

3 large avocados
Juice from 1 lime
2 large Roma tomatoes, diced
2 cloves garlic, minced

¼ cup chopped fresh cilantro
¼ cup chopped red onion
½ teaspoon salt
½ teaspoon freshly ground black pepper

1. Cut avocados in half lengthwise, remove the pit, and scoop them out of the skin and into a medium bowl. Add lime juice. Use a fork to mash avocado and lime together, leaving some chunks intact.
2. Add tomatoes, garlic, cilantro, onions, salt, and pepper. Mash with a fork until combined.

PER SERVING	Fat: 14.1g	Sodium: 303mg	Carbohydrates: 14.3g
Calories: 193	Protein: 3.0g	Fiber: 8.3g	Sugar: 3.0g

Turmeric-Infused Panna Cotta

Turmeric used to be considered an exotic spice, but it is now widely available in any supermarket, even the fresh root version. Try this pungent condiment, and the earthy but distinct flavor will surely win you over.

Makes 6 fat bombs

1½ cups coconut milk, refrigerated and cream separated from the water

1½ cups beef stock

1½ tablespoons powdered unflavored gelatin

1 tablespoon turmeric

½ tablespoon sea salt

1. In a small saucepan over medium heat, heat coconut cream and beef stock.
2. Whisk in gelatin until completely incorporated.
3. Add turmeric and salt and simmer 5 minutes.
4. Pour mixture evenly into 6 small glasses or ramekins.
5. Refrigerate until set, at least 6 hours or overnight.
6. Serve in glass or invert over a small plate after dipping glass into hot water a few seconds.

PER 1 FAT BOMB			
Calories: 98	Fat: 8.1g	Sodium: 710mg	Carbohydrates: 3.1g
	Protein: 2.8g	Fiber: 0.4g	Sugar: 1.7g

Chicken Skin Crisps with Spicy Avocado Cream

Sometimes a bit of spice is a great complement to the creaminess of an ingredient. That makes for a well-balanced recipe.

Makes 6 fat bombs

Skin from 3 chicken thighs
1½ ounces (¼ medium) avocado pulp
1½ ounces sour cream

½ fresh jalapeño pepper, seeded and finely chopped
½ teaspoon sea salt

1. Preheat oven to 350°F. On a cookie sheet, lay out skins as flat as possible.
2. Bake 12–15 minutes until skins turn light brown and crispy, being careful not to burn them.
3. Remove skins from cookie sheet and place on a paper towel to cool.
4. In a small bowl, combine avocado pulp, sour cream, jalapeño, and sea salt.
5. Mix with a fork until well blended.
6. Cut each crispy chicken skin into 2 pieces.
7. Place 1 tablespoon avocado mix on each chicken crisp and serve immediately.

PER 1 FAT BOMB	Fat: 6.0g	Sodium: 204mg	Carbohydrates: 0.8g
Calories: 71	Protein: 2.4g	Fiber: 0.4g	Sugar: 0.3g

Stuffed Chicken Breast

You can use frozen spinach in place of the fresh spinach for this recipe. Just make sure it's completely thawed and drained before use, or the filling will be runny.

Serves 4

1 pound (4 individual) boneless, skinless chicken breasts
¼ cup cream cheese, softened
¼ cup sour cream
1 (10-ounce) package fresh spinach, chopped

⅓ cup chopped fresh basil
1 tablespoon minced green onions
½ cup shredded pepper jack cheese
2 cloves garlic, minced
¼ teaspoon salt
¼ teaspoon freshly ground black pepper

1. Preheat oven to 375°F.
2. Cut a slit into the side of each chicken breast to create a pocket.
3. Combine all other ingredients in a medium bowl and beat until smooth.
4. Fill each chicken breast with ¼ of the mixture and secure pocket closed with toothpicks.
5. Place chicken breasts in a 9" × 13" baking dish and cook for 35 minutes, or until chicken is no longer pink.

PER SERVING
Calories: 271

Fat: 12.7g
Protein: 30.8g

Sodium: 346mg
Fiber: 1.7g

Carbohydrates: 4.7g
Sugar: 1.3g

Creamy Chicken Zoodles

This recipe calls for zucchini noodles, or zoodles, which you can easily make with a vegetable spiralizer. You can find a spiralizer at most home stores. If you prefer, you can also make zucchini noodles by julienning the zucchini with a vegetable peeler.

Serves 4

2 large zucchini

3 tablespoons extra-virgin olive oil

1 pound boneless, skinless chicken breast, cut into cubes

½ teaspoon salt

½ teaspoon freshly ground black pepper

8 ounces fresh spinach

½ cup cream cheese

2 tablespoons grated Parmesan cheese

2 tablespoons feta cheese crumbles

1. Cut zucchini in long strips with a vegetable peeler or a spiralizer. Set zucchini aside on a paper towel and allow to sweat.
2. Heat olive oil in medium skillet over medium heat. Season chicken cubes with salt and pepper and add to hot pan. Cook chicken until no longer pink, about 10 minutes.
3. Remove chicken from pan with slotted spoon and set aside.
4. Add spinach to hot pan and sauté until wilted. Add cream cheese, Parmesan cheese, and feta cheese, and stir until melted. Add chicken back to pan and toss until coated. Remove from heat and pour over zucchini noodles.

PER SERVING

Calories: 383	Fat: 22.8g	Sodium: 600mg	Carbohydrates: 8.5g
	Protein: 31.8g	Fiber: 2.8g	Sugar: 5.0g

Shepherd's Pie

This recipe freezes very well, so save yourself some time by doubling the recipe and freezing half. You can use the frozen pie for dinner on a night when you don't feel like cooking.

Serves 6

2 tablespoons coconut oil
1 medium yellow onion, chopped
3 cloves garlic, minced
2 medium stalks celery, diced
1 medium zucchini, diced
1½ pounds ground lamb
1 teaspoon dried rosemary
1 teaspoon dried thyme

1 teaspoon freshly ground black pepper
½ teaspoon salt
½ teaspoon garlic powder
4 cups cauliflower florets, boiled
¼ cup heavy cream
3 tablespoons unsalted butter
½ teaspoon garlic salt
¾ cup shredded Cheddar cheese

1. Preheat oven to 350°F.
2. Heat coconut oil in a large skillet over medium-high heat. When oil is hot, add onions and garlic and sauté until translucent, about 5 minutes. Add celery and zucchini and sauté until soft, another 5 minutes.
3. Add lamb, herbs, spices, and garlic powder and cook until no longer pink. Pour lamb mixture into a 9" × 13" baking dish.
4. Put boiled cauliflower, cream, butter, and garlic salt in a food processor and process until smooth. Pour cauliflower mixture on top of lamb. Top with cheese.
5. Bake until cheese is melted and pie is bubbly, about 25 minutes. Allow to cool for 10 minutes before serving.

PER SERVING	Fat: 24.9g	Sodium: 531mg	Carbohydrates: 12.2g
Calories: 357	Protein: 20.7g	Fiber: 4.4g	Sugar: 7.1g

Some Shepherd's Pie History
Shepherd's pie, which is also called cottage pie, was first developed in an attempt to use up leftover meat. Traditional shepherd's pie uses lamb. When beef is used instead of lamb, the same meal is called cottage pie.

Meaty Chili

This recipe calls for a mixture of bacon and pork, but you can use any combination of ground meat that you want.

Serves 8

8 slices thick-cut sugar-free bacon
1 medium white onion, chopped
1 large green bell pepper, diced
1 small red bell pepper, diced
1 pound 85/15 ground beef
1 pound ground pork
1 (14.5-ounce) can fire-roasted diced
  tomatoes

1 (6-ounce) can tomato paste
3 tablespoons chili powder
1 tablespoon cumin
1 teaspoon garlic powder
2 teaspoons sugar-free hot sauce
1 teaspoon salt
1 cup sugar-free beef broth

1. Cook bacon over medium-high heat in a large skillet until crisp, about 10 minutes.
2. Remove bacon from heat, reserving bacon fat, and chop into small pieces.
3. Put chopped onions and peppers in the same skillet in hot bacon grease and sauté until translucent, 3–4 minutes. Add ground beef and ground pork and cook until no longer pink. Drain liquid.
4. Put beef mixture, chopped bacon, and remaining ingredients in a slow cooker. Stir until ingredients are combined and cook on low for 6 hours.

PER SERVING	Fat: 17.1g	Sodium: 1,025mg	Carbohydrates: 11.2g
Calories: 292	Protein: 20.8g	Fiber: 3.4g	Sugar: 5.5g

Searching for Sugar
Not all hot sauces are the same. Some of them contain sugar, even though it's not necessary. Check your hot sauce labels and choose one that is sugar-free. A lot of popular brands fall into this category.

Pull-Apart Pork

This is excellent on keto "sandwiches," or served by itself. It also freezes well and can be stored in single-serving containers for quick meals.

Serves 6

1 tablespoon coconut oil
2 pounds pork stew meat, cubed
2 yellow onions, peeled and chopped
4 medium tomatoes, chopped
4 cloves garlic, minced
2 teaspoons chili powder

¼ teaspoon ground cinnamon
¼ teaspoon cayenne pepper
2 teaspoons dried oregano
2 teaspoons ground cumin
½ teaspoon salt
¼ cup apple cider vinegar

1. Melt the coconut oil in a large skillet over medium heat. Sauté the pork and onions in the oil until the meat is lightly browned, about 5–8 minutes.
2. Mix the tomatoes and garlic together in a large bowl.
3. Mix the spices, salt, and vinegar in a small bowl.
4. Place half of the tomato mixture in the bottom of a slow cooker. Sprinkle with ¼ of the spice mixture.
5. Place the meat mixture over the tomato layer, and sprinkle with ½ of the spice mixture.
6. Place the remaining tomato mixture on top of the meat, and sprinkle with the remaining spice mixture.
7. Cover and heat on a low setting for 6–8 hours.

PER SERVING	Fat: 27.0g	Sodium: 324mg	Carbohydrates: 8.0g
Calories: 414	Protein: 27.4g	Fiber: 2.1g	Sugar: 3.6g

Chicken Peanut Stew

Sprinkle with chopped peanuts and flaked coconut before serving over freshly cooked cauli-flower "rice."

Serves 4

4 (4-ounce) boneless, skinless chicken
  breasts
1 large green bell pepper
2 medium yellow onions
1 (6-ounce) can tomato paste
¾ cup unsalted sugar-free crunchy peanut
  butter

3 cups sugar-free chicken broth
1 teaspoon salt
1 teaspoon chili powder
1 teaspoon granulated erythritol or granular
  Swerve
½ teaspoon ground nutmeg

1. Cut the meat into 1" cubes.
2. Remove the stem and seeds from the pepper and cut into ¼" rings. Peel the onions and cut into ¼" rings.
3. Combine all the ingredients in a slow cooker; stir until all ingredients are well mingled.
4. Cover and cook on a low setting for 4–6 hours.

PER SERVING
Calories: 472
Fat: 27.3g

Protein: 38.1g
Sodium: 1,307mg
Fiber: 7.8g

Carbohydrates: 26.1g
Sugar: 11.2g
Sugar alcohol: 1.0g

Lamb Vindaloo

You can also prepare this with pork or beef; the cooking times will stay the same.

Serves 4

¾ cup rice vinegar
¼ cup water
1 teaspoon black peppercorns, roughly pounded
1 tablespoon minced garlic
2 teaspoons chili powder
2 green serrano chilies, minced
1½ pounds boneless lean lamb, cubed

3 tablespoons light olive oil
1 tablespoon grated gingerroot
1 large red onion, peeled and finely chopped
6 whole dried red chilies, roughly pounded
1 (1") cinnamon stick
½ teaspoon turmeric powder
½ teaspoon salt

1. In a slow cooker insert combine the rice vinegar, water, black peppercorns, garlic, chili powder, and green chilies. Add the lamb and coat evenly with the marinade. Refrigerate, covered, for 1 hour.
2. In a deep pan, heat the oil over medium heat. Add the gingerroot and sauté for about 10 seconds. Add the onions and sauté for about 7–8 minutes or until golden brown.
3. Add the dried red chilies, cinnamon stick, and turmeric powder; sauté for 20 seconds.
4. Remove the lamb pieces from the marinade. Add the lamb to the pan with onions and sauté on high heat for about 10 minutes or until the lamb is browned and the oil starts to separate from the mixture.
5. Transfer the browned lamb back to the slow cooker. Mix with the marinade and salt. Cover and cook on high for 4–5 hours, or on low for 8–10 hours, or until the lamb is cooked through and tender. Serve hot.

PER SERVING	Fat: 31.6g	Sodium: 406mg	Carbohydrates: 6.1g
Calories: 426	Protein: 22.8g	Fiber: 1.5g	Sugar: 1.9g

Selecting Lamb

Color can be a great help when buying lamb. Younger lamb is pinkish red with a velvety texture. It should have a thin layer of white fat surrounding it. If the meat is much darker in color, it means that the lamb is older and flavored more strongly.

Creamed Brussels Sprouts

For a cheesier, gooier dish, add ½ cup of shredded Cheddar cheese to these Brussels sprouts before you sprinkle on the pork rinds.

Serves 4

5 tablespoons unsalted butter, divided
2 cloves garlic, minced
2 cups sliced Brussels sprouts
¾ cup heavy cream

2 tablespoons grated Parmesan cheese
¼ teaspoon salt
¼ teaspoon freshly ground black pepper
½ cup crushed pork rinds

1. Preheat oven to 350°F.
2. Heat 2 tablespoons butter in a medium skillet over medium-high heat. Add garlic and sauté for 3 minutes. Add Brussels sprouts and continue to sauté until Brussels sprouts are fork tender, about 5 minutes.
3. Transfer Brussels sprouts, garlic, and melted butter to a 9" × 9" baking dish. Add cream, Parmesan cheese, salt, and pepper. Sprinkle pork rinds evenly over the top of Brussels sprouts and top with remaining butter.
4. Cover and bake for 30 minutes. Serve hot.

PER SERVING			
Calories: 351	Fat: 31.9g	Sodium: 348mg	Carbohydrates: 6.1g
	Protein: 7.7g	Fiber: 1.7g	Sugar: 2.2g

Bacon-Wrapped Asparagus

Don't let the simplicity of this recipe fool you. These Bacon-Wrapped Asparagus stalks are always a crowd pleaser.

Serves 4

12 asparagus spears, ends trimmed   6 slices sugar-free bacon

1. Cut each strip of bacon in half lengthwise.
2. Wrap a piece of bacon around each asparagus spear and secure in place with a toothpick.
3. Grill over medium heat for 10 minutes, or until bacon is crisp, turning each spear over halfway through cooking time.

PER SERVING	Fat: 5.8g	Sodium: 291mg	Carbohydrates: 2.2g
Calories: 90	Protein: 6.9g	Fiber: 1.0g	Sugar: 0.9g

Stuffed Baby Bella Mushroom Caps

Mushrooms make an excellent holder for meat-based fat bombs. These bombs use a hearty and earthy tasting mushroom filled with the proper proportion of tangy cheese and savory sausage.

Makes 8 fat bombs

1 tablespoon extra-virgin olive oil
8 baby bella mushrooms, cleaned and
  stems removed
¼ teaspoon salt

4 ounces pork breakfast sausage, at room
  temperature
4 tablespoons chopped fresh parsley
½ cup shredded Parmesan cheese

1. Preheat oven to 350°F.
2. Rub olive oil on mushroom tops and sprinkle lightly with salt.
3. Mix sausage, parsley, and cheese in a small mixing bowl.
4. Stuff each mushroom cap until mixture forms a nice cap slightly above the mushroom ribbing.
5. Bake on a cookie sheet roughly 20 minutes until sausage becomes browned and cheese browns slightly. Serve warm.

PER 1 FAT BOMB	Fat: 6.8g	Sodium: 257mg	Carbohydrates: 1.7g
Calories: 90	Protein: 5.2g	Fiber: 0.2g	Sugar: 0.5g

Turnip Fries

Turnips are often overlooked at the supermarket, but they make a great alternative to carbohydrate-loaded potatoes when making fries.

Serves 2

2 large turnips, peeled and cut into 2" sticks
2 tablespoons olive oil
4 tablespoons grated Parmesan cheese

¼ teaspoon salt
¼ teaspoon freshly ground black pepper
¼ teaspoon chili powder

1. Preheat oven to 425°F.
2. Place turnip sticks on foil-lined baking pan. Sprinkle olive oil, Parmesan cheese, salt, pepper, and chili powder over turnips and toss to coat. Spread in single layer.
3. Bake in the oven for 15 minutes, flip fries over, and then bake for another 15 minutes. Serve warm.

PER SERVING
Calories: 173

Fat: 12.4g
Protein: 4.2g

Sodium: 578mg
Fiber: 2.8g

Carbohydrates: 11.2g
Sugar: 5.6g

Fried Cauliflower "Rice"

When shredding the cauliflower, process it just enough to create rice-like pieces, but not so much that it begins to blend together. If you process it too long, it will turn into mashed cauliflower.

Serves 6

1 large head cauliflower (about 6 cups)
2 tablespoons unsalted butter
2 tablespoons sesame oil
4 cloves garlic, minced
2 green onions, chopped

2 tablespoons coconut aminos
½ teaspoon garlic salt
3 large eggs, beaten
1 large avocado, sliced

1. Break cauliflower into florets and put through a food processor using the grating attachment.
2. In a large wok or skillet, heat butter and sesame oil. Add minced garlic and sauté on medium for 3 minutes.
3. Add cauliflower and sauté for another 5 minutes, stirring frequently, until cauliflower is softened. Add green onions, coconut aminos, garlic salt, and eggs and toss until eggs are cooked.
4. Top with sliced avocado.

PER SERVING			
Calories: 182	Fat: 13.4g	Sodium: 673mg	Carbohydrates: 9.4g
	Protein: 5.9g	Fiber: 3.8g	Sugar: 2.3g

Chorizo-Stuffed Jalapeños

There is perhaps no better pairing than chorizo with spicy peppers baked into a delicious creamy mound of cheese. The addition of bacon is truly the icing on the cake.

Makes 6 fat bombs

1 tablespoon olive oil

¼ medium yellow onion, peeled and minced

6 ounces pork chorizo sausage

4 ounces cream cheese, softened

3 medium jalapeño peppers, seeded and sliced in half

3 slices sugar-free bacon, sliced in half horizontally

1. Preheat oven to 375°F.
2. Add olive oil to a medium skillet over medium heat and sauté onions 2 minutes. Add chorizo to pan and cook another 3–5 minutes. Drain mixture.
3. In medium mixing bowl, whip cream cheese with hand mixer until smooth. Fold in sausage and onion mixture with a spatula.
4. Stuff each pepper half with sausage mixture.
5. Wrap 1 bacon slice around each stuffed pepper in a spiral motion, covering the cheese mixture underneath.
6. Bake 10–15 minutes or until bacon becomes crispy and cheese mixture underneath bubbles through and turns slightly brown. Serve warm.

PER 1 FAT BOMB	Fat: 18.9g	Sodium: 515mg	Carbohydrates: 2.3g
Calories: 233	Protein: 10.0g	Fiber: 0.3g	Sugar: 1.1g

Why Do Americans Love Jalapeño Poppers?

Although their origin is a bit fuzzy, poppers were speculated to be an American spin-off of the Mexican classic chiles rellenos. Nobody can seem to pinpoint who coined the term "poppers" and decided to batter dip, freeze, and commercialize them in the 1980s, but they have been a popular restaurant staple in California restaurants since at least the 1960s.

Pumpkin Pie Smoothie

Don't confuse pumpkin purée with canned pumpkin pie filling. Pure pumpkin purée contains only the flesh of a pumpkin, while pumpkin pie filling contains sweeteners that increase sugar and carbohydrate content.

Serves 2

½ cup pumpkin purée
1 cup full-fat canned coconut milk
½ teaspoon pumpkin pie spice
¼ large avocado

2 tablespoons coconut oil, melted
¼ teaspoon maple extract
¼ cup unsweetened whey protein powder

1. Put all ingredients in a blender and blend until smooth.
2. Serve cold.

PER SERVING	Fat: 38.1g	Sodium: 35mg	Carbohydrates: 8.1g
Calories: 422	Protein: 12.6g	Fiber: 2.8g	Sugar: 1.2g

Avocado Raspberry Smoothie

Sweet and satisfying, this smoothie makes a great breakfast—or a decadent dessert. Try swapping out the raspberries with blueberries, blackberries, or even cloudberries for a more exotic touch.

Serves 1

¼ medium avocado, peeled and pit removed
¼ cup raspberries
½ cup chopped fresh mint

1 cup heavy cream
2 tablespoons coconut oil, melted
½ cup water

1. Place avocado, raspberries, mint, cream, and coconut oil in a blender and blend until smooth.
2. Add water while blending until desired consistency is reached.

PER SERVING

Calories: 1,134	Fat: 114.0g	Sodium: 95mg	Carbohydrates: 15.2g
	Protein: 6.4g	Fiber: 5.3g	Sugar: 8.1g

Matcha Madness Smoothie

Matcha not only adds antioxidants to this smoothie but also a beautiful green hue. The best-quality matcha powders add a bit of earthy flavor and a subtle sweetness too.

Makes 1 fat bomb

½ (13.5-ounce) can full-fat coconut milk
1 tablespoon powdered unflavored gelatin
2 tablespoons almond butter
1 teaspoon vanilla extract

1 tablespoon matcha
6 drops liquid stevia
4 ice cubes

1. Pour milk and gelatin into a blender and blend to combine.
2. Add remaining ingredients except for ice cubes and blend another minute until well mixed.
3. Place ice cubes into blender and process until smoothie thickens. Serve immediately.

PER 1 FAT BOMB	Fat: 55.0g	Sodium: 137mg	Carbohydrates: 15.3g
Calories: 609	Protein: 16.9g	Fiber: 4.0g	Sugar: 1.5g

Coconut Cream Dream Smoothie

Coconut cream pie is a delicious dessert, but it packs empty calories and very few vitamins and minerals. This recipe blends the star ingredients of coconut cream pie in a healthy green smoothie.

Serves 4

1 cup chopped romaine lettuce
Flesh of 2 mature coconuts
1 tablespoon lemon juice
1 medium avocado, peeled and pit removed

¼" piece gingerroot, peeled
½ cup full-fat canned coconut milk
½ cup full-fat plain Greek-style yogurt
1 cup ice cubes

1. Combine romaine, coconut flesh, lemon juice, avocado, gingerroot, and coconut milk in a blender until thoroughly combined.
2. Add the yogurt while blending until just combined.
3. Slowly add ice while blending until desired texture is reached.

PER SERVING
Calories: 844

Fat: 74.3g
Protein: 10.6g

Sodium: 56mg
Fiber: 20.5g

Carbohydrates: 35.9g
Sugar: 13.9g

Banana Nut Smoothie

This smoothie combines ample protein and the healthy fats you need. In addition to the vitamins, minerals, and nutrients from the lettuce and banana the healthy fats from the coconut milk make this smoothie a powerful start to any day.

Serves 4

1 cup full-fat canned coconut milk
1 cup chopped iceberg lettuce
1 cup heavy cream
½ teaspoon vanilla extract

1 cup unsweetened vanilla almond milk, divided
1 medium banana, sliced

1. Combine coconut milk, lettuce, heavy cream, and vanilla extract in a blender with ½ cup almond milk and blend thoroughly.
2. Continue adding remaining almond milk while blending until desired consistency is reached.
3. To serve, divide smoothie into 4 glasses. Top each glass with an equal amount of sliced banana.

PER SERVING
Calories: 353

Fat: 32.9g
Protein: 3.1g

Sodium: 71mg
Fiber: 0.9g

Carbohydrates: 10.5g
Sugar: 5.6g

Caffeine-Free Coconut Vanilla Tea

A hot drink that is a breakfast in itself, this recipe does not have caffeine or dairy, so it is suitable for the strictest of diets.

Makes 1 fat bomb

1 tea bag rooibos tea
1½ cups hot water
2 teaspoons granulated erythritol or granular Swerve

1 tablespoon coconut oil
⅛ teaspoon vanilla extract

1. Place tea bag in water and brew about 8 minutes.
2. Place brewed tea in a blender with remaining ingredients.
3. Blend on high 15 seconds.
4. Serve immediately.

PER 1 FAT BOMB		
Calories: 120	Protein: 0.0g	Carbohydrates: 8.5g
Fat: 12.8g	Sodium: 2mg	Sugar: 0.1g
	Fiber: 0.0g	Sugar alcohol: 8.0g

Po Cha (Tibetan Butter Tea)

Tibetan Butter Tea is originally made with yak butter and a potent brew of smoky tea leaves. You do not have to look for yak butter to re-create this flavorful drink at home; you'll still reap all the benefits of starting your day off right with a high-fat treat.

Makes 2 fat bombs

4 cups water
2 tablespoons black tea leaves
2 tablespoons unsalted butter

2 tablespoons heavy cream
⅛ teaspoon sea salt
1 drop smoke flavor

1. In a small saucepan over high heat bring water to a boil, then lower heat to low.
2. Add tea leaves to water and simmer about 3 minutes. Strain.
3. Combine brewed tea with remaining ingredients in a blender and mix on high about 3 minutes.
4. Serve immediately.

PER 1 FAT BOMB			
Calories: 157	Fat: 16.0g	Sodium: 241mg	Carbohydrates: 1.9g
	Protein: 0.4g	Fiber: 0.0g	Sugar: 0.4g

The Original Recipe

This Tibetan recipe is a staple of their culture. Po Cha is consumed every day, multiple times a day. The drink has many benefits, including giving warmth to the drinker and providing a stable, long-lasting energy source, which is much needed at high altitudes.

Thai Iced Coffee

Every Thai restaurant serves some version of this drink. Now you can enjoy this version, which is full of beneficial fat.

Makes 2 fat bombs

4 cups strong brewed coffee, cooled

4 teaspoons granulated erythritol or granular Swerve

2 tablespoons full-fat canned coconut milk

⅛ teaspoon vanilla extract

4 tablespoons heavy cream

1. Pour coffee into a large bowl and mix with sweetener, coconut milk, and vanilla extract.
2. Pour coffee mixture over ice in 2 tall glasses. Pour cream on top of coffee without stirring, so layers remain separate.
3. Serve immediately with a tall spoon and a straw.

PER 1 FAT BOMB		
Calories: 138	Protein: 1.5g	Carbohydrates: 9.3g
Fat: 13.6g	Sodium: 21mg	Sugar: 0.9g
	Fiber: 0.0g	Sugar alcohol: 8.0g

Chocolate Brownie Cheesecake

Throw a handful or two of nuts into this recipe to increase the unsaturated fat content and make this dessert even more nutritious.

Serves 12

4 ounces unsweetened chocolate
½ cup unsalted butter
4 large eggs, divided
2¼ cups granulated erythritol or granular
    Swerve, divided
1½ teaspoons vanilla extract, divided

½ cup almond flour
½ teaspoon salt
16 ounces cream cheese, softened
¼ cup sour cream
¼ cup full-fat canned coconut milk

1. Preheat oven to 325°F.
2. Melt chocolate and butter together in a medium saucepan over low heat.
3. In a large bowl, beat 2 eggs, 1½ cups granulated erythritol or Swerve, and 1 teaspoon vanilla extract until combined. Add almond flour and salt. Beat until incorporated. Add chocolate and butter mixture and beat until smooth.
4. Pour brownie mixture into the bottom of a greased 9" springform pan.
5. Bake for 20 minutes, or until a knife inserted in the center of the brownies comes out clean, then remove and reduce oven temperature to 300°F.
6. Beat cream cheese in a stand mixer until fluffy, about 2 minutes.
7. Add sour cream and coconut milk and beat until incorporated. Beat in remaining 2 eggs, remaining ¾ cup granulated erythritol or Swerve, and remaining ½ teaspoon vanilla extract.
8. Pour cream cheese mixture over brownie mixture.
9. Bake for 45 minutes. Let cool and store in refrigerator until ready to serve.

PER SERVING	Protein: 6.0g	Carbohydrates: 41.7g
Calories: 324	Sodium: 167mg	Sugar: 1.6g
Fat: 28.0g	Fiber: 2.1g	Sugar alcohol: 36.0g

Peanut Butter Cookies

Give these cookies a crunch by using crunchy peanut butter instead of creamy peanut butter or by adding a few handfuls of chopped peanuts.

Serves 18

1 cup sugar-free peanut butter
¼ cup unsalted butter, softened
1 cup granulated erythritol or granular
   Swerve

1 large egg, lightly beaten
1 teaspoon vanilla extract
½ teaspoon baking soda
¼ teaspoon sea salt

1. Preheat oven to 350°F.
2. In a medium mixing bowl, beat together peanut butter and butter until combined and fluffy.
3. Add granulated erythritol or Swerve, egg, and vanilla extract and mix until combined.
4. Stir in baking soda and salt.
5. Drop by tablespoonfuls onto an ungreased cookie sheet.
6. Bake for 10 minutes, or until lightly browned.

PER SERVING		
Calories: 111	Protein: 3.9g	Carbohydrates: 13.8g
Fat: 9.7g	Sodium: 71mg	Sugar: 0.9g
	Fiber: 1.3g	Sugar alcohol: 10.8g

Chocolate Ice Cream

This recipe calls for the use of an ice cream maker, but not having one isn't a deal breaker. Instead of using an ice cream maker, you can stir the mixture in the bowl every 30–45 minutes while it cools in the refrigerator.

Serves 4

1 large ripe avocado
1 cup full-fat canned coconut milk
1 cup heavy cream
1 teaspoon vanilla extract

1 cup unsweetened cocoa powder
1 cup granulated erythritol or granular
   Swerve

1. Cut avocado in half and scoop out contents into a medium bowl, excluding the pit. Add coconut milk, heavy cream, and vanilla extract to the bowl. Beat mixture until smooth.
2. Add cocoa powder and granulated erythritol or Swerve and beat until smooth.
3. Store in a metal bowl in the refrigerator for 6–12 hours, then put mixture into an ice cream maker, following manufacturer's instructions for use.
4. Serve immediately or store in the freezer until ready to serve.

PER SERVING		
Calories: 425	Protein: 7.2g	Carbohydrates: 66.8g
Fat: 39.7g	Sodium: 36mg	Sugar: 2.3g
	Fiber: 10.3g	Sugar alcohol: 48.7g

Make It Your Own

This is a basic ice cream recipe that you can make your own by adding your own mix-ins. Try unsweetened coconut flakes, dark chocolate shavings, or chopped peanuts.

Raspberries and Cream Panna Cotta

A heavenly dream of flavor with real raspberries and cream, sure to uplift anyone's day. Give it a try!

Makes 2 fat bombs

1 cup heavy whipping cream

1 teaspoon powdered unflavored gelatin

1 tablespoon granulated erythritol or granular Swerve

⅛ teaspoon raspberry flavor

2 tablespoons freeze-dried raspberries

1. Pour cream into a small saucepan, sprinkle gelatin on top, and let sit 5 minutes.
2. Add sweetener and raspberry flavor to saucepan.
3. Place saucepan over low heat and whisk until ingredients are well blended, about 3 minutes.
4. Simmer over very low heat about 1 minute, stirring constantly.
5. Pour into 2 glasses or molds. Sprinkle dried raspberries equally over glasses or molds.
6. Refrigerate until set, at least 6 hours or overnight.
7. Serve in glass or invert over a small plate after dipping glass into hot water a few seconds.

PER 1 FAT BOMB		
Calories: 426	Protein: 5.6g	Carbohydrates: 10.4g
Fat: 41.8g	Sodium: 51mg	Sugar: 3.9g
	Fiber: 0.3g	Sugar alcohol: 6.0g

Coconut Custard

This is a perfect variation of the famous custard, suitable for people with dairy sensitivities. You will find it so delicious, though, that it will become a well-loved recipe for everyone.

Makes 2 fat bombs

1 cup coconut cream
1 large egg
1 large egg yolk
½ cup granulated erythritol or
   granular Swerve

½ teaspoon vanilla extract
½ teaspoon rum extract

1. Preheat oven to 300°F.
2. Place 2 ramekins in a deep baking pan just large enough to hold them.
3. In a small saucepan over low heat bring coconut cream to a simmer.
4. In a small bowl whisk together remaining ingredients until eggs are foamy and sweetener is dissolved.
5. Slowly pour egg mixture into coconut cream, whisking constantly to combine well.
6. Pour mixture through a fine strainer into ramekins, using a spoon to help you.
7. Pour hot water into baking pan halfway up ramekins.
8. Bake until custard is set, about 35 minutes.
9. Remove from oven and let cool in baking pan about 4 hours.
10. Can be stored in refrigerator up to 3 days.

PER 1 FAT BOMB		
Calories: 305	Protein: 4.5g	Carbohydrates: 52.6g
Fat: 28.3g	Sodium: 59mg	Sugar: 4.3g
	Fiber: 0.0g	Sugar alcohol: 48.0g

Almond Pistachio Fudge

This delightful fudge is full of nutty goodness. The addition of firm coconut oil and coconut milk helps give this fudge body and texture. You'll find ghee, or clarified butter, at most larger markets or online.

Makes 12 fat bombs

¼ cup cocoa butter
½ cup almond butter
½ cup coconut oil
¼ cup full-fat canned coconut milk, chilled overnight

2 tablespoons ghee
2 teaspoons vanilla extract
⅛ teaspoon salt
¼ cup chopped pistachios

1. Grease and line an 8" × 8" baking pan with parchment paper.
2. Melt cocoa butter in a small saucepan over low heat and set aside.
3. In a large bowl add all ingredients except nuts and melted cocoa butter. Mix with a hand mixer until texture is fluffy.
4. Pour melted cocoa butter into almond mixture and combine with hand mixer on low speed.
5. Spread mixture evenly into pan and sprinkle with pistachios.
6. Refrigerate at least 4 hours to set. Cut into 12 bars and serve from refrigerator.

PER 1 FAT BOMB	Fat: 22.8g	Sodium: 58mg	Carbohydrates: 3.3g
Calories: 226	Protein: 3.0g	Fiber: 1.6g	Sugar: 0.6g

Pizza Balls

This recipe takes the ultimate Italian dish and magically transforms it into a fat bomb. Whenever the urge for pizza hits you, reach for this instead.

Makes 6 fat bombs

2 ounces fresh mozzarella

2 ounces cream cheese

1 tablespoon olive oil

1 teaspoon tomato paste

6 large kalamata olives, pitted

12 fresh basil leaves

1. In a small food processor, process all ingredients except basil until they form a smooth cream, about 30 seconds.
2. Form mixture into 6 balls, with the aid of a spoon.
3. Place 1 basil leaf on top and bottom of each ball and secure with a toothpick.
4. Serve immediately or refrigerate up to 3 days.

PER 1 FAT BOMB	Fat: 7.6g	Sodium: 193mg	Carbohydrates: 1.1g
Calories: 91	Protein: 2.7g	Fiber: 0.4g	Sugar: 0.5g

Kalamata Olive and Feta Balls

This recipe brings you the flavors of Greece on a warm sunny day by the Mediterranean Sea.

Makes 6 fat bombs

2 ounces cream cheese
2 ounces feta cheese
12 large kalamata olives, pitted

⅛ teaspoon finely chopped fresh thyme
⅛ teaspoon fresh lemon zest

1. In a small food processor, process all ingredients until they form a coarse dough, about 30 seconds.
2. Scrape mixture and transfer to a small bowl, then refrigerate 2 hours.
3. Form mixture into 6 balls, with the aid of a spoon.
4. Serve immediately or refrigerate up to 3 days.

PER 1 FAT BOMB	Fat: 6.0g	Sodium: 307mg	Carbohydrates: 1.5g
Calories: 77	Protein: 1.9g	Fiber: 0.7g	Sugar: 0.7g

Spicy Bacon and Avocado Balls

These fat bombs carry some of the flavors of guacamole. They are slightly spicy, but if you want to increase the fire, just leave some of the jalapeño seeds in.

Makes 6 fat bombs

4 slices sugar-free bacon
1 medium avocado, pitted and peeled
2 tablespoons coconut oil
1 tablespoon bacon fat
1 tablespoon finely chopped green onions

2 tablespoons finely chopped fresh cilantro
1 small jalapeño pepper, seeded and finely chopped
¼ teaspoon sea salt

1. In a medium skillet over medium heat, cook bacon until golden, about 4 minutes each side.
2. Drain bacon on a paper towel. Save bacon fat for later in a glass cup.
3. Once bacon is cool, chop 2 slices into crumbles.
4. Cut remaining 2 slices into 3 pieces each; these will be the bases for your fat bombs.
5. Smash avocado with a fork in a small bowl.
6. Add coconut oil and cooled bacon fat to avocado.
7. Add onions, cilantro, jalapeño, salt, and bacon crumbles. Blend well with a fork.
8. Refrigerate a minimum 30 minutes.
9. Form mixture into 6 balls, with the aid of a spoon.
10. Place remaining 6 bacon pieces on a plate, then top each with an avocado ball.
11. Serve immediately or refrigerate up to 3 days.

PER 1 FAT BOMB			
Calories: 132	Fat: 12.0g	Sodium: 230mg	Carbohydrates: 2.3g
	Protein: 3.1g	Fiber: 1.6g	Sugar: 0.2g

Cocoa Coconut Butter Fat Bombs

In addition to coconut oil, this recipe uses coconut butter, which differs from the oil. Coconut butter is the puréed meat of mature coconuts, while coconut oil has been separated from the coconut meat. One cannot be substituted for the other.

Makes 12 fat bombs

1 cup coconut oil
½ cup unsalted butter
6 tablespoons unsweetened cocoa powder

15 drops liquid stevia
¾ cup coconut butter

1. Add coconut oil, butter, cocoa powder, and stevia to a small saucepan over medium-low heat. Stir frequently until all ingredients are melted, about 2 minutes.
2. Melt coconut butter in a separate small saucepan.
3. Pour 2 tablespoons of cocoa mixture into each well of a 12-cup silicone mold.
4. Add 1 tablespoon of melted coconut butter to each well.
5. Place in the freezer until hardened, about 30 minutes.
6. Store in the refrigerator.

PER 1 FAT BOMB	Fat: 31.3g	Sodium: 4mg	Carbohydrates: 4.2g
Calories: 303	Protein: 1.3g	Fiber: 2.3g	Sugar: 0.7g

Cinnamon Bun Fat Bombs

These Cinnamon Bun Fat Bombs have the same flavor as a cinnamon roll fresh from the oven, but without the sugar and carbohydrates.

Makes 12 fat bombs

1 cup coconut butter, softened
¼ teaspoon plus ⅛ teaspoon ground cinnamon, divided

¼ teaspoon ground nutmeg
¼ teaspoon vanilla extract
¼ cup crushed walnuts

1. Combine coconut butter, ¼ teaspoon cinnamon, nutmeg, and vanilla extract in a small bowl and mix until well combined.
2. Separate the mixture into 12 equal parts and roll into ball shapes. Place on a cookie sheet lined with wax paper.
3. Mix crushed walnuts with remaining cinnamon in a small bowl. Roll balls in nut mixture until coated.
4. Place finished balls back on the cookie sheet lined with wax paper and refrigerate until ready to eat.
5. Store in the refrigerator.

PER 1 FAT BOMB	Fat: 14.9g	Sodium: 6mg	Carbohydrates: 5.8g
Calories: 163	Protein: 1.7g	Fiber: 2.9g	Sugar: 1.4g

Smooth It Out
The crushed walnuts finish off these fat bombs with a nice crunch, but you could also grind the walnuts instead for a smooth, but still decadent, finish.

Maple Fat Bombs

These Maple Fat Bombs provide comforting maple flavor, without all of the carbohydrates contained in regular maple syrup.

Makes 12 fat bombs

¼ cup unsalted butter
½ cup coconut butter
10 drops liquid stevia

½ teaspoon maple extract
¼ teaspoon ground cinnamon
½ cup crushed walnuts

1. Place butter, coconut butter, stevia, maple extract, and cinnamon in a small saucepan and stir over medium heat until melted. Mix thoroughly.
2. Remove mixture from heat and stir in crushed walnuts.
3. Fill each well of a 12-cup mini muffin pan lined with cupcake wrappers or a silicone mold with an equal amount of the mixture.
4. Place pan or mold in the freezer until mixture hardens, about 30 minutes.
5. Store in the refrigerator.

PER 1 FAT BOMB	Fat: 13.3g	Sodium: 3mg	Carbohydrates: 3.4g
Calories: 139	Protein: 1.5g	Fiber: 1.7g	Sugar: 0.8g

Choosing Your Maple

There are four different types of maple extract: pure, natural, imitation, and artificial. Imitation and artificial extracts are made in a lab and often contain no real maple product at all. Stick to pure or natural extracts.

White Chocolate Pecan Fat Bombs

This classic fat-bomb recipe is easy to make and incredibly delicious. Walnuts would be a great substitution if you're out of pecans.

Makes 8 fat bombs

¼ cup pecans
4 tablespoons cocoa butter
4 tablespoons coconut oil

¼ teaspoon vanilla extract
5 drops liquid stevia

1. Chop pecans coarsely with a knife or process quickly in a food processor so they don't get too fine.
2. In a small saucepan over very low heat, add cocoa butter and coconut oil, stirring until completely melted, about 3 minutes.
3. Remove from heat and stir in pecans, vanilla extract, and stevia.
4. Pour into 8 silicone molds.
5. Refrigerate until hard.
6. Remove from mold. Serve immediately or store in refrigerator for up to 1 week.

PER 1 FAT BOMB			
Calories: 140	Fat: 15.0g	Sodium: 0mg	Carbohydrates: 0.5g
	Protein: 0.3g	Fiber: 0.3g	Sugar: 0.2g

Appendix

Keto Shopping List

The following is a list of keto-approved foods that you should stock your kitchen with during your keto diet. It may even help to bring this list along to the grocery store when you are just starting out on your keto journey. Having a handy guide will help you stay on target with your nutrition.

Fats and Oils

- Butter
- Coconut oil
- Coconut butter
- Olive oil
- Olives
- Avocados
- Avocado oil
- Coconut flakes (unsweetened)
- Full-fat coconut milk

Protein

- Poultry: chicken, turkey, duck (free-range is best)
- Meat: beef, veal, venison, bison, lamb (grass-fed is best)
- Pork: pork loin, ham, pork chops (humanely treated, pastured is best; make sure ham contains no sugar)
- Eggs
- Bacon
- Sausage
- Deli meat: prosciutto, pepperoni, turkey, roast beef, ham (make sure there is no added sugar)
- Fresh fish: cod, salmon, halibut, mackerel, herring, sardines, tuna, anchovies (wild-caught is best)

- Shellfish: shrimp, crab, lobster, scallops, mussels, oysters, clams
- Canned tuna
- Canned salmon

Dairy Products

- Heavy cream
- Sour cream
- Ricotta cheese
- Cottage cheese
- Cream cheese
- Cheddar cheese
- Parmesan cheese
- Pepper jack cheese
- Mozzarella cheese
- Asiago cheese

Fruits

- Blackberries
- Blueberries
- Raspberries
- Granny Smith apples
- Lemons

Vegetables

- Bell peppers
- Cucumbers
- Broccoli
- Eggplant
- Spinach
- Baby kale

- Cabbage
- Cauliflower
- Lettuce (iceberg and romaine)
- Onions
- Garlic
- Scallions
- Shallots
- Mushrooms
- Celery
- Brussels sprouts
- Asparagus
- Zucchini
- Spaghetti squash
- Canned whole tomatoes
- Fire-roasted diced tomatoes

Nuts, Nut Butters, and Seeds

- Almonds
- Almond butter
- Cashews
- Cashew butter
- Pecans
- Pistachio nuts
- Macadamia nuts
- Chia seeds
- Peanuts
- Peanut butter
- Walnuts
- Pumpkin seeds
- Sunflower seeds

Condiments

- Pickles
- Mustard
- White vinegar
- Apple cider vinegar
- Hot sauce

Sweeteners, Extracts, and Miscellaneous

- Erythritol (granulated and powdered)
- Stevia (liquid and granulated)
- Vanilla extract
- Almond extract
- Orange extract
- Peppermint extract
- Pork rinds
- Dark chocolate
- Unsweetened cocoa powder
- Whey protein powder (sugar-free—low net carbohydrates)

US/Metric Conversion Chart

VOLUME CONVERSIONS	
US Volume Measure	Metric Equivalent
⅛ teaspoon	0.5 milliliter
¼ teaspoon	1 milliliter
½ teaspoon	2 milliliters
1 teaspoon	5 milliliters
½ tablespoon	7 milliliters
1 tablespoon (3 teaspoons)	15 milliliters
2 tablespoons (1 fluid ounce)	30 milliliters
¼ cup (4 tablespoons)	60 milliliters
⅓ cup	90 milliliters
½ cup (4 fluid ounces)	125 milliliters
⅔ cup	160 milliliters
¾ cup (6 fluid ounces)	180 milliliters
1 cup (16 tablespoons)	250 milliliters
1 pint (2 cups)	500 milliliters
1 quart (4 cups)	1 liter (about)
WEIGHT CONVERSIONS	
US Weight Measure	Metric Equivalent
½ ounce	15 grams
1 ounce	30 grams
2 ounces	60 grams
3 ounces	85 grams
¼ pound (4 ounces)	115 grams
½ pound (8 ounces)	225 grams
¾ pound (12 ounces)	340 grams
1 pound (16 ounces)	454 grams

OVEN TEMPERATURE CONVERSIONS

Degrees Fahrenheit	Degrees Celsius
200 degrees F	95 degrees C
250 degrees F	120 degrees C
275 degrees F	135 degrees C
300 degrees F	150 degrees C
325 degrees F	160 degrees C
350 degrees F	180 degrees C
375 degrees F	190 degrees C
400 degrees F	205 degrees C
425 degrees F	220 degrees C
450 degrees F	230 degrees C

BAKING PAN SIZES

American	Metric
8 × 1½ inch round baking pan	20 × 4 cm cake tin
9 × 1½ inch round baking pan	23 × 3.5 cm cake tin
11 × 7 × 1½ inch baking pan	28 × 18 × 4 cm baking tin
13 × 9 × 2 inch baking pan	30 × 20 × 5 cm baking tin
2 quart rectangular baking dish	30 × 20 × 3 cm baking tin
15 × 10 × 2 inch baking pan	30 × 25 × 2 cm baking tin (Swiss roll tin)
9 inch pie plate	22 × 4 or 23 × 4 cm pie plate
7 or 8 inch springform pan	18 or 20 cm springform or loose bottom cake tin
9 × 5 × 3 inch loaf pan	23 × 13 × 7 cm or 2 lb narrow loaf or pâté tin
1½ quart casserole	1.5 liter casserole
2 quart casserole	2 liter casserole

Index